Shahin Nikmanzar
Alireza Tabib Khoei
Sarehnaz Aghili

Surgical and Superficial Anatomy of the Head and Neck

Shahin Nikmanzar
Alireza Tabib Khoei
Sarehnaz Aghili

Surgical and Superficial Anatomy of the Head and Neck

Noor Publishing

Imprint
Any brand names and product names mentioned in this book are subject to trademark, brand or patent protection and are trademarks or registered trademarks of their respective holders. The use of brand names, product names, common names, trade names, product descriptions etc. even without a particular marking in this work is in no way to be construed to mean that such names may be regarded as unrestricted in respect of trademark and brand protection legislation and could thus be used by anyone.

Cover image: www.ingimage.com

Publisher:
Noor Publishing
is a trademark of
Dodo Books Indian Ocean Ltd., member of the OmniScriptum S.R.L Publishing group
str. A.Russo 15, of. 61, Chisinau-2068, Republic of Moldova Europe
Printed at: see last page
ISBN: 978-620-3-85878-5

Surgical and Superficial Anatomy of the Head and Neck

By

MD. Shahin Nikmanzar

Neurosurgeon

Dr. Alireza Tabib Khoei

Neurosurgeon, Faculty Member and Associate, Professor of Iran
University of Medical Sciences

Dr. Sarehnaz Aghili

Obstetrics and Gynecology Resident

MD Shahin Nikmanzar

Neurosurgeon

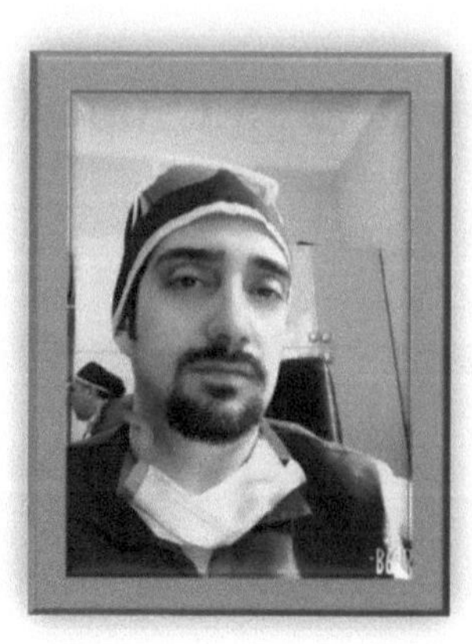

Dr. Alireza Tabib Khoei

Neurosurgeon, Faculty Member and Associate,
Professor of Iran University of Medical Sciences

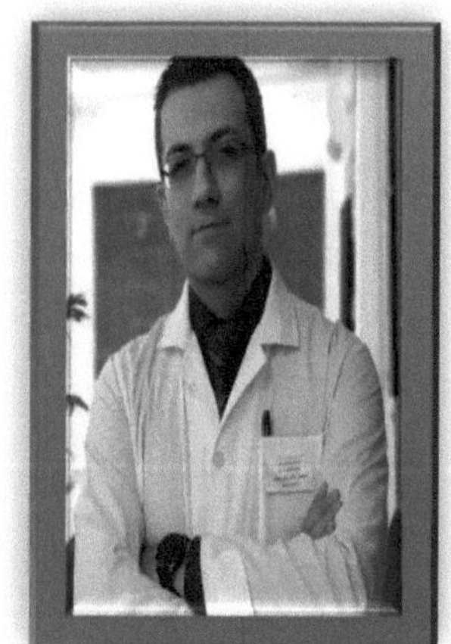

Dr Sarehnaz Aghili

Obstetrics and Gynecology Resident

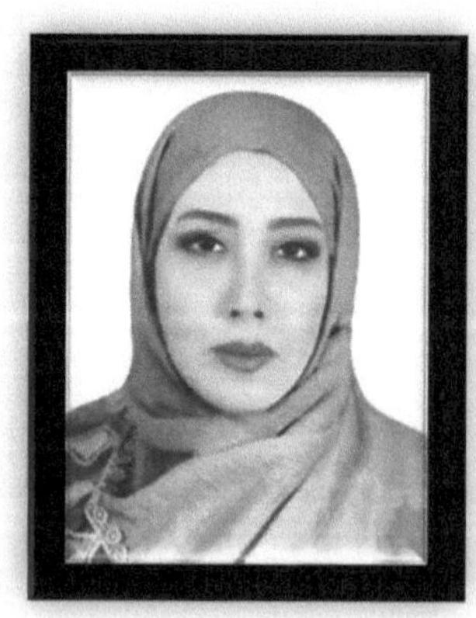

This Book is dedicated to

My Family's

Content

Chapter I

Superficial Anatomy of the Neck

Introduction

The neck is the area between the head and torso and its boundaries are:

A) Above

1) Symphysis menti

2) Base of mandible

3) Mastoid process

4) Superior nuchal line

5) External occipital protuberance

B) At the bottom

1) Supra sternal or jugular notch

2) Clavicle

3) Acromion

4) A line that connects the acromion of the two sides so that it passes through the thorny appendage of the seventh cervical vertebra (C_7).

The neck is divided into the following two parts:

1) Posterior or Back of the neck: The part of the neck that is covered by the trapezius muscles.

2) Antero lateral: From the front sides of the trapezius muscles to the midline is called the outer front. The back of the neck is examined in the back (Back) and in this part the external front is examined.

Neck bone symptoms

Symphysis menti

In the midline, where the two halves of the mandible are connected, it can be felt as an indistinct ridge.

Inferior border or base of mandible

It extends from the symphysis menti to the mandibular angle and is easily palpable.

Mandibular angle

It is located between the lower side of the mandible and the back of the mandible (Ramus) and is located at the level of the second cervical vertebra (C_2) and is easy to touch.

Mastoid process

It is located behind the ear and is easy to touch. In infants, this appendage does not develop and grows with head movements and muscle stretching.

External occipital protuberance

It is in the middle behind and the most prominent part of it is called Inion.

Superior nuchal line

It extends from the external occipital ridge to the mammary appendage, and the Trapezius and Sternocleidomastoid (SCM) muscles attach to this line.

Hyoid bone

It is the only independent bone in the neck that is located at the level of the third cervical vertebra (C_3) and is in the shape of a horseshoe whose body and large cornua are palpable. To touch its body in the anatomical position, go down about one centimeter from the chin (Symphysis menti) and then press back with your hand, in which case the body of the bone is touched, which is a good sign to find the site of laryngeal anesthesia. If you inject anesthetic into the lower part of the big horn, the upper part of the laryngeal vocal cords will be anesthetized.

In addition, the tip of the great horn near the anterior side of the SCM muscle is important in locating the lingual artery in surgery and is in the middle of the line that connects the laryngeal protrusion (Adam's apple) to the mammary appendage of the temporal bone. To touch this part, first relax the neck and then touch the tip of the big horn by holding one side steady.

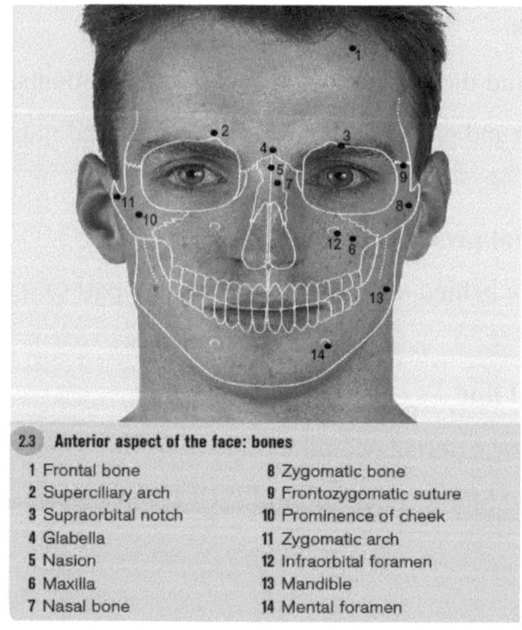

Figure 1. Anterior aspect of the face bones

Suprasternal or jugular notch

It can be felt as a depression at the lower end of the midline of the neck and above the sternum (Manubrium of sternum). It is located at the level of the second thoracic vertebra in men and the third thoracic vertebra (T_3) in women.

Sternoclavicular joint

On the outside, the incision is located above the chin and in the space between the two joints of the SCM muscle, and by moving the shoulder up and down, the joint surface is touched, which is an important sign in the head, neck and trunk.

Clavicle: It can be felt all over.

Acromion: It can be touched above the shoulder and at the end of the clavicle.

Transverse extensions of the cervical vertebrae: If a person turns his head slightly to one side and in this case draw a line from the apex of the temporal bone to the middle of the clavicle on the same side, the transverse extensions of the cervical vertebrae are on this line in the following order and may be palpable.

1) **Transverse process of the atlas vertebra (C_1):** In the distance between the apex of the mammary gland and the angle of the mandible may be touched and at the beginning of the spinal cord, there is a large

hole of the occipital bone (Foramen magmum) and hard palate (Hard palate).

2) The transverse process of the second cervical vertebra (C_2) or Axis may be felt at the level of the mandibular angle on the line and deep in the SCM muscle.

3) Transverse appendage of the third cervical vertebra (C_3): Located on the upper surface of the hyoid bone (Hyoid) and deep in the SCM muscle.

4) Transverse appendage of the fourth cervical vertebra (C_4): Located on the incision surface of the thyroid cartilage.

5) Transverse appendage of the fifth cervical vertebra (C_5): It is level with the middle part of the thyroid cartilage and is located behind the SCM muscle.

6) Transverse appendage of the sixth cervical vertebra (C_6): It is on the surface of the lower lateral cartilage of the ring (Cricoid). On the anterior surface, this appendage has a protrusion called the carotid tubercle, on which the common carotid artery can be pressed and the pulse of the artery can be touched. This appendage is just above the midpoint of the clavicle.

7) Transverse appendage of the seventh cervical vertebra (C_7): It is located behind the clavicle and therefore is not touched and is located at the level of the isthmus (Isthmus) of the thyroid gland and is the highest point of the thoracic duct.

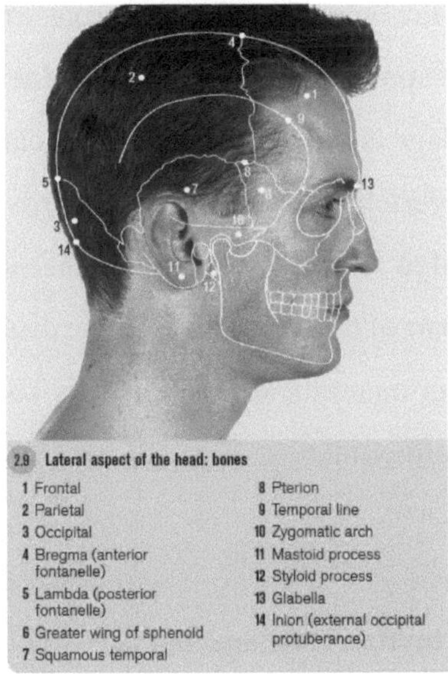

Figure 2. Lateral aspect of the head bones

Symphysis menti

Hyoid bone

It is located at the level of the third cervical vertebra (C_3) and indicates the beginning of the larynx.

Thyrohyoid membrane

It is a membrane that stretches between the lamina and the upper side of the thyroid cartilage and can be felt as a depression between the two signs.

Thyroid cartilage

The largest cartilage of the larynx is in the form of a shield and has two blades (Lamina) that are connected at the front and create a laryngeal prominence or Adam's apple, which is more prominent and clearer in men. The notch of this cartilage is next to the top of this cartilage and at the level of the fourth cervical vertebra (C_4). The vocal cords attach to the back of this cartilage. This bulge is easily felt and if the person bends his head backwards, the upper part of this cartilage is in the distance between the chin and the sternum, but in anatomical position it is closer to the chin. This cartilage moves by swallowing.

Cricoid cartilage

It is located below the thyroid cartilage and is easily below the bulge of the palpable larynx. This cartilage is an important superficial sign because its lower side is level with the following points:

I.   Sixth cervical vertebra (C_6)

II.   The junction of the larynx with the trachea

III.   The junction of the throat with the esophagus

IV.   The surface where the vertebral artery enters the transverse hole of the sixth cervical vertebra (C_6).

V.   The surface at which the inferior thyroid artery enters the thyroid gland and the middle thyroid vein exits.

VI.   Middle cervical sympathetic ganglion

VII.   The surface on which the superior ventricle of the omohyoid muscle passes over the carotid sheath.

VIII.   The place where the carotid artery can be pressed on the carotid tubercle of the transverse appendage of the sixth cervical vertebra (C_6) and the pulse of the artery can be touched.

(Emergency membrane) Cricothyroid membrane or ligament

It is located as a depression between thyroid and cricoid cartilage and is palpable.

All the palpable structures above the larynx are the larynx (Larynx) and should be gently touched. In some cases, a foreign body may become trapped at the entrance to the laryngeal inlet or in the space between the true vocal cords (Rima glottidis), blocking the airway and causing suffocation, and it may also occur.

The foreign body gets stuck in the laryngeal sinus and trachea or bronchi, causing glottic spasm and suffocation. Inflammation of the upper larynx (for example, in diphtheria or chickenpox) may also cause swelling of the mucosa by effusion of fluid into the loose submucosal tissue (Oedema of glottis), resulting in suffocation.

Fluid infiltration does not occur under the vocal cords, as the mucosa is firmly attached to the vocal cords. In cases where the airway is closed, the larynx or trachea should be opened by cutting the superficial layers. In very urgent cases, the cricothyroid membrane is cut with a small transverse incision and a tube is inserted into the lower part of the larynx, which is called a laryngotomy.

First ring of trachea

It is felt under the thyroid cartilage.

Isthmus of thyroid gland

On the second, third and sometimes fourth ring, it covers the trachea and is touched as a soft object under the hand.

Lower tracheal rings

They are located below the thyroid gland and are further away from the skin, but may be felt with deeper pressure.

Jugular notch

It is also T_2 level in men and T_3 level in women.

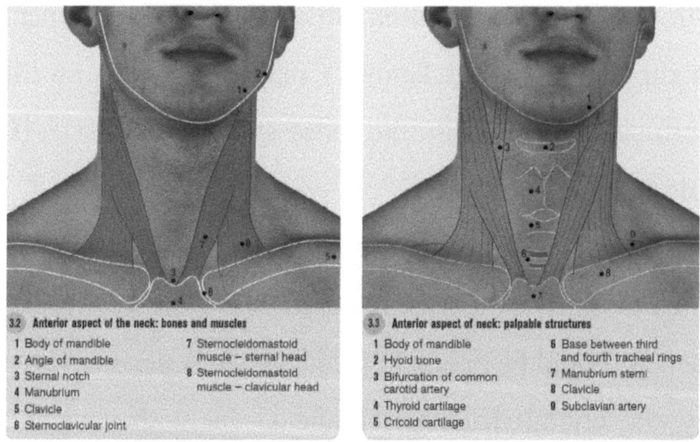

Figure 3. Anterior aspect of the neck

Tracheostomy

In emergencies, and especially when more space is needed to stay airway, they use this technique, which has two types, upper and lower.

Superior tracheostomy

In this case, a vertical incision is made in the skin under the cricoid cartilage, and after pushing the muscles, the thyroid gland is lowered and the second and third rings of the trachea are cut and a special tube is inserted into the trachea. In this case, there is a possibility of damage to the jugular venous arch.

Inferior tracheostomy

The incision is made at the top of the incision above the sternum. After raising the thyroid gland, a longitudinal incision is made in the fourth and fifth rings of the trachea and a special tube is inserted into the trachea will have. In addition, this type of tracheostomy is difficult and dangerous to create in children because the neck is short and the Left brachiocephalic vein may rise to the top of the sternal incision. The opening of the airway should be completely in the midline.

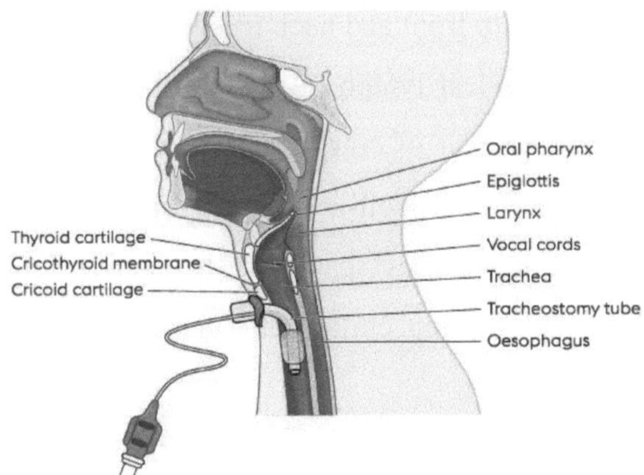

Figure 4. Lateral view of the neck

Muscles that can be felt and seen in the neck

Neck skin muscle (Platysma)

The thin muscle is equivalent to the fly muscle (Panniculus carnosus) in some mammals, which extends from the chest to the lower jaw and is part of the facial expression muscles. When a person tries to turn their lower jaw to one side or pull the corner of their lip down (the way they are used to make faces and shave their faces), the muscle fibers are identified and in the case of contraction of the lateral muscles These muscles are also identified.

Sternocleidomastoid muscle (SCM)

It is one of the obvious surface signs in the neck, which is clearly characterized by bending the neck to one side and turning the face to the opposite side, and especially creating resistance to this action. This muscle has two clavicle and external ends at the bottom, which create a triangular space between these two ends, which is known as the Lesser supraclavicular fossa. In this cavity is the Sternoclavicular joint. This muscle divides the outer front of the neck into front and back triangles.

Inflammation of the cervical lymph nodes (Cervical lymphadenitis) puts pressure on the eleventh pair of cranial nerves, the spinal accessory, and consequently the cortex (Torticolli), especially in children. In addition, central nerve stimulation causes spasm of this muscle and neck. Also, bleeding in this muscle during childbirth can cause congenital torticolli muscle and neck shortening.

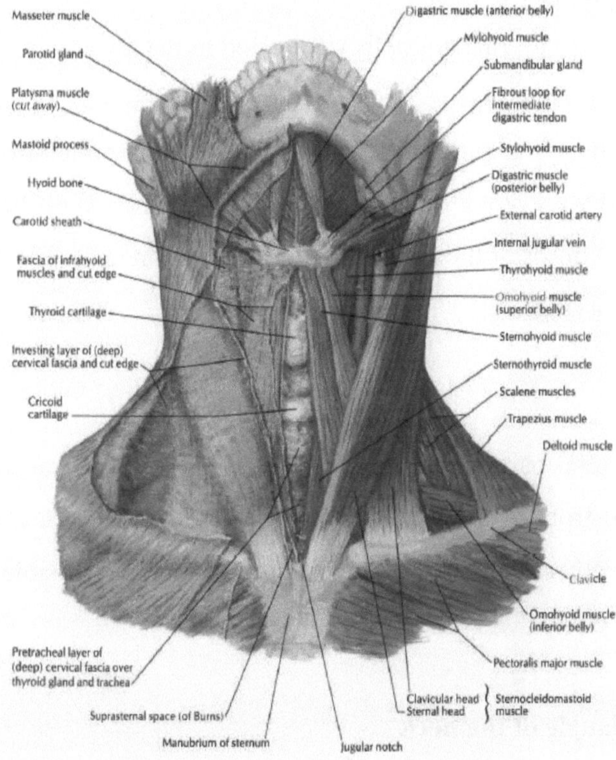

Figure 5. Muscles in the Neck

Trapezius muscle

The anterior side of this muscle extends from the superior nuchal line to the third of the clavicle in the neck and is marked and visible by raising the shoulder against the resistance of the anterior side. The anterior side of this muscle forms the dorsal side of the dorsal triangle of the neck.

Omohyoid muscle

The lower ventricle (Inferior belly) is located in the lower part of the dorsal triangle of the neck and is felt and seen above the clavicle and may be confused with a lymph node or a mass. This muscle is pulled from the SCM muscle at the level of the cricoid cartilage to the junction of the outer third and inner two thirds of the clavicle, and if the person raises his shoulders, it is marked as a ridge.

Neck areas

The anterolateral part of the neck is divided by the SCM muscle into two triangles, the front and the back of the neck. These triangles, in turn, are divided into other triangles by other muscles, here only visible and tactile triangles are given.

Anterior triangle of the neck

Its top is at the bottom and its sides are:

A) Inside: Midline.

B) Outside: The front side of the SCM muscle.

C) Above (base): The lower side of the mandible.

Back triangle of neck

This triangle is not completely behind the neck, but on the outer surface of the neck and behind the SCM muscle. The apex of this triangle is about 4 cm behind the ear. Its sides are:

A) In front: SCM back muscle.

B) In the back: the front side of the Trapezius muscle.

C) At the bottom: the middle third of the clavicle.

The lower part of this triangle is clearer and is known as the Greater Supracalvicular Fossa.

Submental region

This area or triangle is located between the chin and the lamina, and the floor of this triangle is formed by the mylohyoid muscle. There are several lymph nodes in this cavity, which drain the lymph from the tip of the tongue and the lower lip, and during herpes, these nodes become swollen.

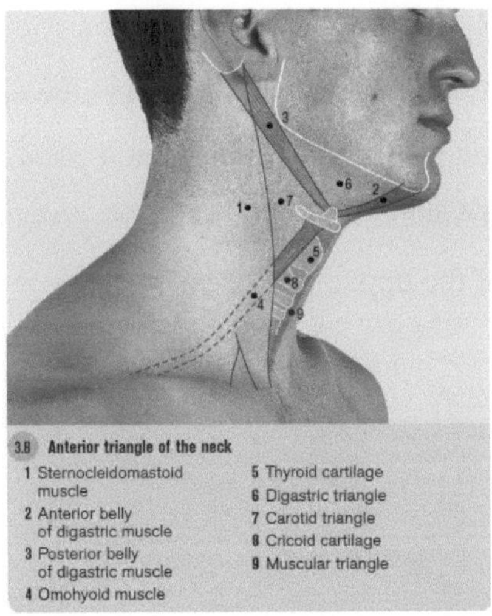

Figure 6. Anterior triangle of the neck

Glands that can be felt and seen in the neck

Thyroid gland

Glands weighing 25 grams and H-shaped, which has two lobes, right and left, and isthmus (Isthmus). The upper limit of the gland is at the level of the fifth cervical vertebra (C_5) and the lower limit is at the level of the first thoracic vertebra (T_1). Each thyroid lobe is about 5 cm long and 3 cm wide and covers the second and third rings of the trachea. To determine the surface path of each part, proceed as follows:

Strait (Isthmus): Draw two transverse lines 1.25 cm long and 1.25 cm apart so that the transverse line is about one centimeter below the cricoid cartilage.

Upper pole: Connect the following points to get the upper pole:

A) On the anterior side of the SCM muscle at a point that is flush with the middle of the larynx (Adam's apple).

B) At the outer end of the upper side of the gorge

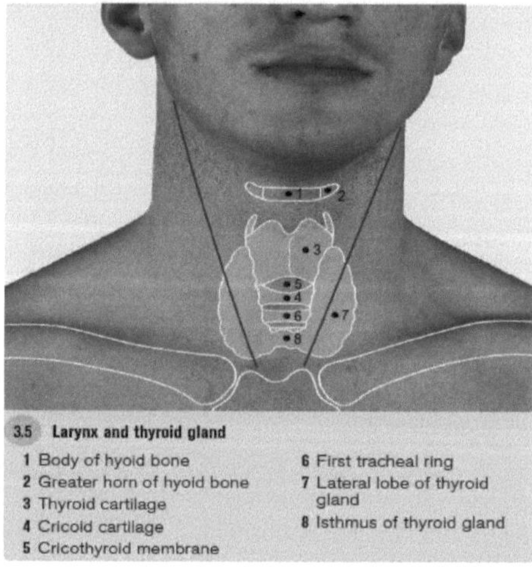

Figure 7. Larynx and thyroid gland

ower pole of each lobe: Connect the following points (albeit with a convexity downwards).

A) One centimeter below the lower side of the gorge

B) Two centimeters outside point a

The thyroid gland is a soft tissue, but it is usually palpable and visible. To view the gland, one must bend one's head back slightly and drink some water, in which case the movement of the gland and the symmetry of the two lobes can be observed. Cricoid cartilage is a good sign to touch the thyroid gland. When swallowing, the gland under your hand is touched. Women have larger and more flexible thyroid than men. Any type of enlarged thyroid gland is called a goiter.

Submandibular or submaxillary salivary gland

It has two parts, surface and depth. To show the surface position, connect the following points so that an oval is obtained:

I. At the mandibular angle

II. Right in front of the front side of the muscle (Masseter)

III. 1.5 cm above the lower edge of the mandible between two points A web

IV. On the large horn (Greater cornua) of the lamina bone

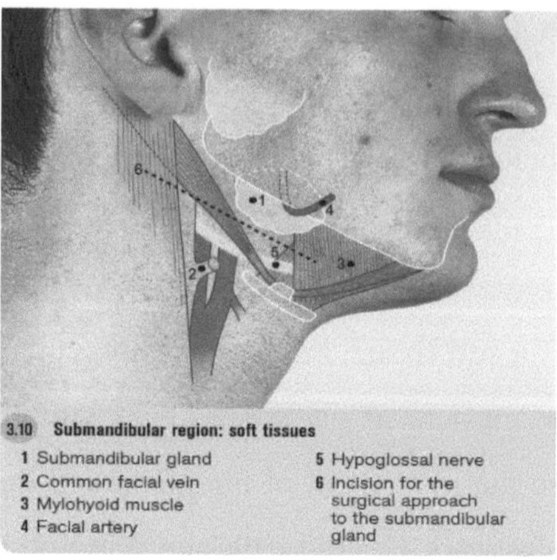

Figure 8. Submandibular region

Its superficial part can be touched in front of the mandibular angle with a careful examination, and if the lymph nodes in this area become large, they can be touched on it. To feel the depth, place the index finger in the floor of the mouth and the thumb in the front and inside the angle of the mandible below the floor of the mouth. The duct of this gland (Warton duct) in the floor of the mouth on both sides of the tongue frenulum can be felt and seen as a sublingual papilla.

Arteries of the Neck

The main arteries of the neck are the subclavian and common carotid arteries, although each of these arteries supplies blood to other areas such as the upper limbs, trunk, head, brain, and spinal cord. How these two arteries separate is different on the right and left. The right arteries arise from the bifurcation of the brachiocephalic trunk. The location of these two branches is at the level of the right sternoclavicular joint. On the left side of each of these two branches originate separately from the aortic arch inside the chest. The path inside the thoracic and left brachiocephalic arteries was examined in the thoracic section, and the cervical path of the right and left arteries is similar. In this section, first the path of the arteries and then the place of touching the pulse of that artery or pressing the artery to prevent bleeding is examined.

Subclavian artery

By connecting the following points together, a curve is obtained, which is convex upwards and shows the path of the artery:

A) Sternoclavicular joint.

B) The midpoint of the clavicle.

C) Two centimeters above the clavicle in the distance between points A and B.

The pulse of this artery can be felt above the midpoint of the clavicle and pressed against the first rib.

Common carotid artery

By connecting the following points, its surface path is determined:

A) Sternoclavicular joint.

B) The anterior side of the Sternocleidomastoid muscle on the upper lateral surface of the thyroid cartilage.

This artery is mostly covered deep in the SCM muscle. At point B, it develops an enlargement known as the carotid sinus. It is then divided into internal and external carotid branches. This sinus has a blood pressure receptor (Barroreceptor) that stimulates and touches it to reduce blood pressure and heart rate. Carotid pulse may be visible if you look at the front and inside of the SCM muscle. The common carotid pulse, because it is closer to the heart (especially on the right side), shows the aortic pulse more accurately. To feel the pulse of this artery, it is better to take it below the upper side of the thyroid cartilage and with the thumb pulse (in general, using the thumb to pulse the large arteries is more useful). The carotid pulse should not be taken bilaterally, as this may interfere with the blood supply to the brain in some people. The common carotid artery usually has no branches in the neck except for the two end branches.

Internal carotid artery

It is relatively deep and its surface path is determined by connecting the following points:

A) on the SCM muscle near its anterior side at a level equal to the upper side of the thyroid cartilage.

B) On the intertragic notch, the earlobe is at the level of the mandibular neck. At this point, the artery enters the skull. Because this artery passes close to the ear, it can be heard in the ear during sleep.

External carotid artery

By connecting the following points, its path can be obtained on the surface:

A) The anterior side of the SCM muscle on the upper lateral surface of the thyroid cartilage

B) The distance between the nipple of the mastoid process (mastoid process) and the angle of the mandible inside the parotid behind the neck of the mandible. At point B, it divides into two terminal branches, the maxillary arteries and the superficial temporal arteries.

In general, a large number of arteries are taken above the upper side of the thyroid cartilage, and it is not possible to determine which artery the pulse belonged to.

The external carotid artery in the neck has branches, the detachment and path of each of which are examined separately.

Superior thyroid artery: By connecting the following points together, its superficial path is determined:

A) The anterior side of the external carotid artery at the bottom of the Greater cornua.

B) Upper pole of the thyroid gland.

Lingual artery

Near and at the level of the tip of the great horn of the lamina bone is separated and spoken.

Facial artery

Its path in the neck is obtained by connecting the following points:

A) Just above the great horn of the lamina.

B) The width of one finger above the front of the mandible angle.

C) The anterior side of the masseter muscle near the lower side of the mandible. At point B, it is located deep in the salivary gland and at point C, its pulse can be taken. The arteries of the face in the neck and face are spiral.

Occipital artery

Above the great horn of the lamina and in the opposite direction, the facial artery separates from the external carotid and goes to the occipital region. The pulse of this artery can be felt behind the mastoid process of the temporal bone.

Posterior auricular artery

It separates slightly above the occipital artery and travels backwards.

Thyroid artery ima

If present, it separates from the trunk of the brachiocephalic artery and travels in front of the trachea to reach the isthmus (Isthmus) of the thyroid gland. This artery may rupture at inferior tracheostomy and cause severe bleeding.

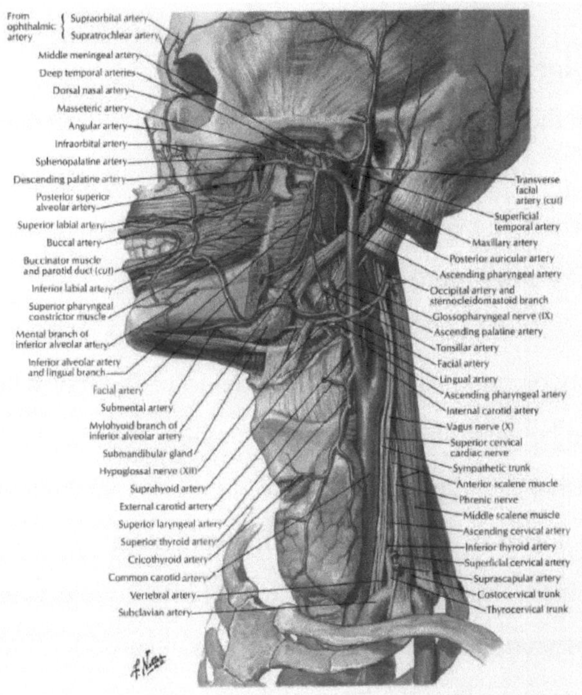

Figure 9. Arteries of the head and neck

Veins of the Neck

It consists of deep veins and two superficial veins on each side.

Subclavian vein

By connecting the following points by a wide strip with a convexity upwards, its path is obtained:

A) Right inside the midpoint of the clavicle

B) The inner side of the clavicle (Clavicular head) of the SCM muscle or Sternoclavicular joint

Internal jugular vein

By connecting the following points, its surface path is determined by a wide bar:

I.   From the soft area (Lobule) of the ear or Intertrgic notch

II.   Sternoclavicular joint

This vein has two upper and lower bulbs, the lower bulb of which is located in the distance between the external and clavicle ends of the SCM muscle or the upper cavity of the small clavicle (Lesser supraclavicular fossa), in which there is a pair of valves has it. This vein receives various branches, including the facial, venous, superior, and middle thyroid veins, where the middle thyroid vein passes through the common carotid at the level of the cricoid cartilage and enters the internal dorsal vein.

External jugular vein

The surface position of the vein is determined by connecting the following points:

A) Slightly below and behind the angle of the mandible inside the parotid gland.

B) The midpoint of the back of the SCM muscle.

C) Slightly inside the midpoint of the clavicle.

This vein is superficial and has a valve at the end, but these valves do not prevent blood from returning. Because the superior vena cava (SVC) and brachiocephalic veins do not have valves, contraction (systole) of the right atrium causes a wave of dilation toward these arteries, causing a weak pulse at the root of the neck in the external jugular vein. pulse) This pulse becomes more pronounced in right heart failure or in tricuspid stenosis. The vena cava and pulse of the valves below 12 are seen as problems. Of course, the internal jugular vein also has a pulse that is somewhat difficult to detect and requires more experience.

Anterior jugular vein

It forms near the lamina bone and descends between the midline and the anterior side of the SCM muscle. At the bottom of the neck, it passes deep into the muscle and drains into the external vena cava or under the clavicle. The anterior jugular vein connects the two sides at the top of the incision above the chin and forms the jugular arch. This vein is visible in the upper two thirds of the neck and may be damaged in the inferior tracheostomy. In general, the jugular veins are clearer when exhaling against resistance (or when crying, such as valves).

Measurement of central venous pressure (CVP)

In many cases, central venous pressure measurement, which indirectly reflects right atrial pressure, cardiac output, and blood volume, is necessary. To do this, a special tube (catheter) is inserted into one of the veins near the heart, i.e. the internal vestibule or under the clavicle (preferably on the right side) and the pressure of the said vein is measured.

The following two places are suitable for inserting the needle into the internal jugular vein

1) In the midpoint of the anterior side of the SCM muscle outside the carotid pulse. At this point, the needle should be inserted into the back of the muscle and outward so as not to damage the surrounding arteries.

Inside the upper cavity of the small clavicle (Lesser supraclavicular fossa): first the external head of the SCM muscle is pulled inwards and then the needle is inserted in the downward direction and into this space.

B) In the case of a vein, the subclavian needles can be inserted into the inner third of the clavicle from above or below the clavicle, and the best place to connect the inner third and outer thirds of the clavicle. If you insert the needle from above, the needle should be on the outside of the SCM muscle, downwards and inwards, while if you want to enter from the bottom of the clavicle, the needle should be inwards and upwards. However, you must keep in mind that the vein is located behind the clavicle.

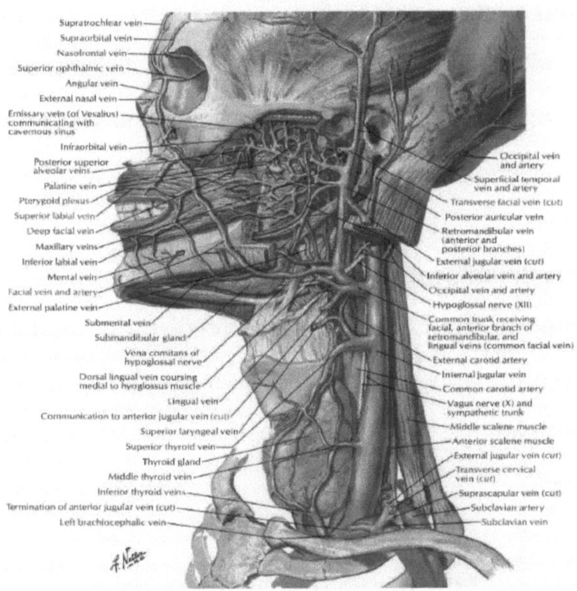

Figure 10. Veins of the head and neck

Lymph nodes of the Neck

Lymph nodes are not normally touched, but become enlarged and palpable due to infection or cancer of the organ receiving the lymph. For this reason, knowing the location of the lymph nodes is important and necessary. Use your index and middle fingertips to touch the lymph nodes. Lymph nodes in the neck are divided into two groups: deep and superficial:

Superficial lymph nodes

Submental nodes

The lymph of the lower lip receives the floor of the mouth and the tip of the tongue, and in herpes these nodules become large and swollen and are located below the chin in the submental triangle.

Submandibular nodes

They are located below the base of the mandible and receive the lymph of the tongue and mouth. These nodules are smaller and softer than the salivary gland.

Parotid or preauricular nodes

They are located in front of the ear and receive the forehead lymph, the temporal region, the upper half of the eardrum, the eyelids and the cheek skin (these nodules are related to the head but were examined in this section).

Nodes on the back of the phone (Retroauricular)

They are located on the surface of the temporal bone and receive the soft lymph of the ear, the floor of the external ear canal, and the skin of the mandible.

Occipital nodes

They are located at the upper angle of the dorsal triangle of the neck and receive the scalp lymph.

Anterior cervical nodes

It is located along the anterior vena cava.

Superficial cervical nodes

It is located along the external jugular vein.

Supraclavicular nodes

It is located deep in the angle created by the clavicle and the SCM muscle, and the enlargement of these nodes on the left is a possible sign of metastasis from a malignancy inside the chest or abdomen.

Deep lymph nodes of the neck

They mainly consist of two groups of upper and lower neck depths:

Superior deep cervical nodes

They are located deep in the SCM muscle and the largest of these is known as the Jugulodigastric node or Tonsilar node.

Inferior deep cervical nodes

They are located mainly deep in the SCM muscle and the largest of them is known as Juguloomohyoid, which is mainly related to the lymphatic system. These nodes are located along the dorsal side of the SCM muscle and the upper nodes are mostly on the front side of the SCM muscle.

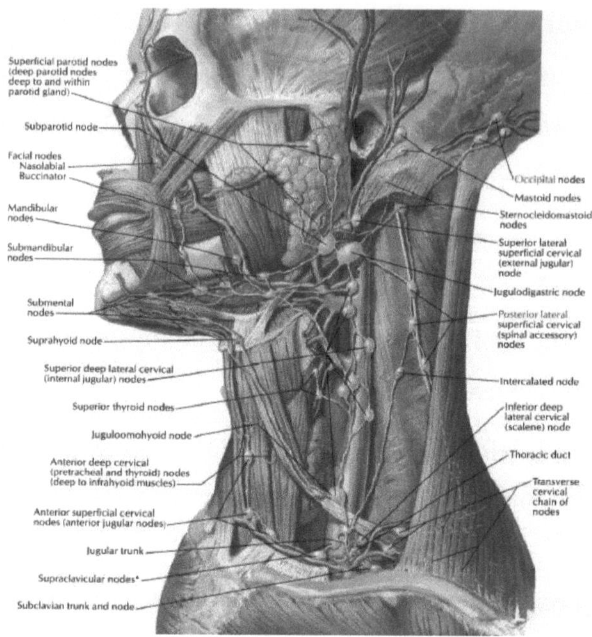

Figure 11. Lymph nodes in the head and neck

Nerves of the Neck

It includes the sympathetic cranial nerves and the cervical and arm nerves, some of which pass through the neck only and have no branches.

Vagus nerve

It has a deep path in the neck and branches to the larynx, throat, heart, ears and meninges. Its surface path is determined by connecting the following points:

A) Intertragic notch in the earlobe (which is about 2 cm deep in this incision).

B) Sternoclavicular joint

One of the branches of the vagus nerve that separates in the neck is the superior laryngeal nerve, which after separation is divided into external and internal branches. The external laryngeal branch is also the path of the upper thyroid artery and gives nerves to the cricothyroid muscle, but the branch of the internal larynx is sensory and after piercing (Thyrohyoid membrane) gives nerves to the mucosa above the vocal cords. To anesthetize this branch of the vagus nerve, anesthesia must be injected under the Greater Cornu. Damage to the vagus nerve or its branches can lead to a wide range of symptoms in the patient. Also, a special examination should be performed to test each branch of the vagus, but in general, hoarseness in vocal cord paralysis and hoarseness in soft palate paralysis can be related to damage to the vagus nerve. To test the vagus nerve while looking at the soft palate, ask him to say the word Aah.

Spinal accessory

This nerve innervates the Sternocleidomastoid and Trapezius muscles, and its superficial path is obtained by connecting the following points:

A) Front and bottom of the earlobe

B) The midpoint between the apex of the mastoid process and the angle of the mandible (on the transverse process of the atlas vertebra)

C) Slightly above the midline of the dorsal side of the SCM muscle

D) About 5 cm above the clavicle on the anterior side of the Trapezius muscle

To test this nerve, place your hands on the person's branches and ask him to raise his shoulders. Central stimulation of this nerve causes muscle spasm and torticollis (Torticolli).

Hypoglossal twelfth pair nerve

It gives nerves to the muscles of the tongue except the palatoglssus. If you connect the following points, the superficial path of the nerve will be determined:

A) Right in front of the Intertragic notch

B) Slightly behind the mandibular angle

C) Slightly above the large horn of the lamina

D) on the lower side of the mandible below the angle of the mouth

To test this nerve, a person must pronounce the word la-la and be able to stick his tongue directly out of his mouth. If the sublingual nerve is damaged on one side, it will deviate to the affected nerve when the tongue is removed.

Cervical sympathetic trunk

The sympathetic trunk or neck chain consists of three ganglia (upper, middle, and lower ganglia) that are connected by fibers. In most cases, the inferior cervical ganglion combines with the first sympathetic ganglion to form the cervicothoracic or stellate ganglion. Connect the following two points to determine the superficial path or sympathetic trunk:

A) Right in front of the Intertragic notch

B) Sternoclavicular joint

All three sympathetic nodes of the neck are located on the line and the location of each on the skin is as follows:

Superior cervical ganglion

It is the largest sympathetic ligament of the neck. To determine the location of this nodule, draw an oval on the surface of the body at a distance between the angle of the upper jaw and the large horn of the lamina on the upper line. This knot is located on the surface between the second and third vertebrae of the neck (C_2-C_3).

Middle cervical ganglion

It is the smallest cervical ganglion and is located on the upper line at the level of the cricoid cartilage and the sixth cervical vertebra (C_6).

Inferior cervical ganglion

It is located on the upper line in the midpoint between the cricoid cartilage and the sternoclavicular joint and in the space between the two ends of the SCM muscle (i.e. in the Lesser supraclavicular fossa).

In some diseases, such as vasospasm of the upper and intracranial limbs, injection into the stellate or cervical-thoracic ganglia relieves pain. To do this, insert the anesthetic into the space between the two ends of the SCM muscle with a needle or place the electrode in the space between the two ends of the muscle for electrical stimulation.

Cervical plexus

Ventral rami form the first to fourth nerves of the neck ($C_1 - C_4$) and has superficial and deep branches, the superficial branches of which are cutaneous and the deep branches are more muscular. In this section, the surface path of different branches of the cervical network is examined:

Deep branches of cervical retina

It includes the branches connecting with different nerves, the muscular branches, the cervical arch (Ansa cervicalis) and the phrenic, in which only the superficial pathway of the phrenic nerve is examined:

Phrenic nerve

It originates from the third, fourth, and fifth nerves of the cervix (C_3-C_4-C_5) and mainly from the fourth nerve (C_4). Gives parts of the pleura and peritoneum. Its surface path is obtained by connecting the following points by a line:

A) At a distance of 4 cm from the midline level with the upper edge of the thyroid cartilage

B) Sternoclavicular joint

How to anesthetize or electrically stimulate a nerve: First pull the Clavicular head of the SCM muscle forward and the midline, then push the needle or electrode toward the anterior tubercle of the transverse appendage of the sixth cervical vertebra (C_6).

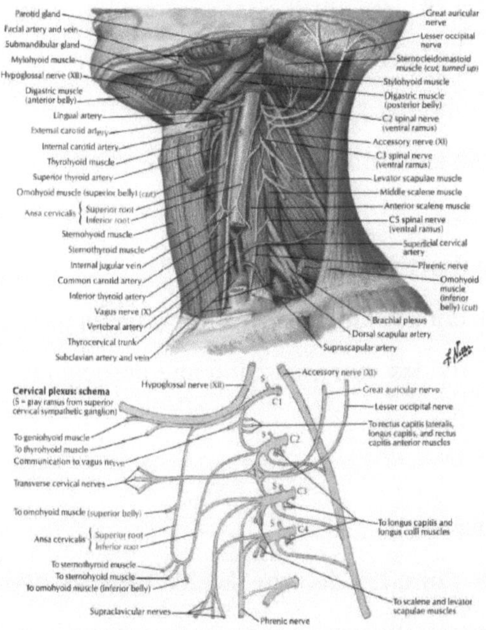

Figure 12. Neural network of the neck

Superficial branches of cervical retina

All superficial branches of the cervical retina become superficial from the midpoint of the dorsal SCM muscle or nerve point.

Lesser occipital nerve

From the midpoint of the dorsal side of the SCM muscle, it travels along the dorsal side of the muscle and supplies the skin on the mammary gland of the temporal bone and the inner surface (cranial) of the eardrum.

Great auricular nerve

After appearing on the back of the SCM muscle, it travels along the external jugular vein and connects to the skin on the parotid gland and the angle of the mandible and the eardrum.

Transverse cervical nerve

After bypassing the dorsal side of the SCM muscle in its midpoint, it crosses to the midline and divides into ascending and descending branches, giving nerve to the skin of the neck.

Supraclavicular nerves

After exiting the dorsal side, the SCM muscle divides into three branches: anterior, middle, and dorsal, and innervates the skin above the chest up to the level of the second rib and on the shoulder. Sometimes the branches of this nerve can be touched on the clavicle under the skin.

How to anesthetize the superficial nerves of the cervical network: Inject the anesthetic into the midline of the back of the SCM muscle. In this case, you should be careful of the external jugular vein or inject the anesthetic separately at the transverse appendage of the cervical vertebrae.

Greater occipital nerve

This nerve separates from the dorsal ramus of the second cervical nerve (C_2) and connects the skin behind the head to the highest part of the skull (Vertex). This nerve can be felt at the point between the mastoid process and the midline. Sometimes pressure on this nerve (for example, when lying on the floor or on a hard pillow) causes pain in the back of the head. This nerve can be anesthetized at this point.

Brachial plexus

The fifth to eighth nerves of the neck (C_5-C_8) and the first thoracic nerve (T_1) are formed by the connection of the anterior branches (Ventral rami) and its trunks are located in the posterior triangle of the neck and after passing through Behind the clavicle, they enter the axillary cavity. The upper torso and to some extent the middle torso of this network are palpable and even visible by tilting the neck to one side and turning the head to the other. In surface anatomy, this network has two sides, upper and lower. By connecting points, A and B, the surface path of the upper side and then by connecting points P and T, the path of the lower side of this network in the neck will be obtained:

    I. The junction of the middle and lower third of the back of the SCM muscle

    II. Just below the tip of the Coracoid scapula

    III. at the angle between the clavicle and the dorsal side of the SCM muscle

    IV. One centimeter below the apex of the Coracoid scapula

How to anesthetize the brachial plexus: The brachial plexus can be anesthetized in the neck and armpits (how to anesthetize the armpit in the upper limb). First get the midpoint of the clavicle by taking the pulse of the subclavian artery. Then inject the needle about two inches above the midpoint of the clavicle. In this injection, you must be very careful that the needle does not enter the lungs. To prevent this complication, it is better to inject a little higher because the injection inside the fascia sheath causes the anesthesia to spread rapidly to the lower areas.

Cervical Dermatomes

The first cervical nerve (C_1) has no cutaneous branch. The second cervical nerve (C_2) usually innervates the skin behind the scalp from the top of the head (vertex) to the superior nuchal line and all the outer surface of the ear and skin at the angle of the mandible. The third cervical nerve (C_3) innervates a thin strip of skin behind the scalp and above the neck across the neck to the midline from the lamina to the first rib. The fourth cervical nerve (C_4) innervates the upper half of the back of the neck and the neck and shoulders.

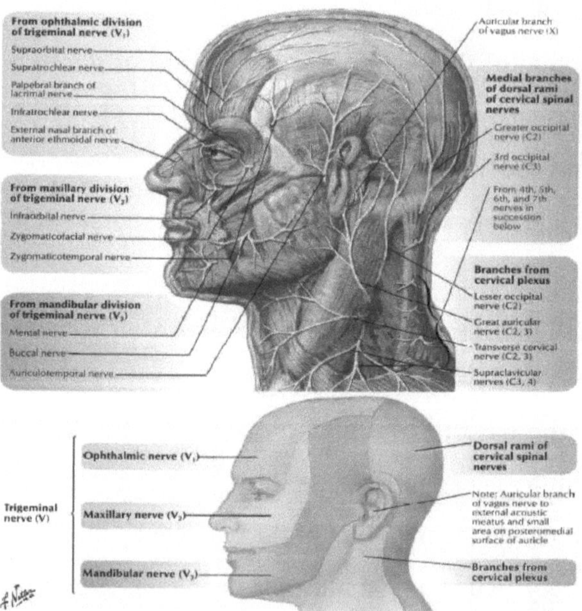

Figure 13. Nerve distribution and cervical nerve nerves

Chapter II

Superficial Anatomy of the Head

Face

It is an area of the head that is limited from the top to the hairline, from the bottom to the chin and from the sides to the earlobe. Due to the interference in speech and expression of facial expressions is the most important factor in identifying and communicating, and the science of aesthetics has a special emphasis on this organ and is important in various other aspects such as psychology, forensic medicine and art. The shape of the face depends not only on the skeleton of the face but also on the arrangement of soft tissues under the skin.

Facial proportions

Usually, any disproportion in the proportions of the face area is easily recognizable. For someone like Leonardo da Vinci, facial proportions are just as important as other body proportions. As these ratios are especially important for plastic surgeons and any other artist. The following is based on Leonardo da Vinci's observations:

In infants, the eyes are located in the middle of the face, but in adults, the eyes are closer to the top of the face and the ratio of the eyes to the top of the face is one third and to the chin is two thirds. In other words, the eyes in the adult are located in the middle of the height of the head.

The width of the two eyes should be equal to each other, the distance between the two eyes and the width of the lower part of the nose. The width of the resting mouth should be equal to the distance between the irises of the eyes. The top of the earlobe should be at the level of the eyebrows and between the eyebrows (Glabella). The upper end of the ear helix (Crus of helix) is at the level of the nasal root (Nasion) while the tip of the nose is at the level of the soft ear (Lobule). The crease between the lower lip and the chin should be approximately at the distance between the tip of the nose and the chin and at the same level as the angle of the mandible.

Many face sizes follow the Rule of thumb, the distance between the tip of the thumb and the metacarpophalangeal joint, which include:

    I. Height of the ear

    II. The distance from the ear to the outer corner of the eye

    III. From the outer angle of the eye to the midline (so the width of the face is equal to 4 thumbs)

    IV. The distance of the hair row to the root of the nose

    V. The distance from the root of the nose to the tip of the nose

    VI. The distance from the tip of the nose to the chin (so the height of the face is equal to three to the thumbs)

    VII. The distance between two irises

The distance between the earlobe (lobule) and the angle of the mandible is equal to half of the thumb. In addition, the height of the face is said to be equal to the length of the palm, which is not so reliable.

Facial types

There are generally two types of face:

    1) Leptoprospic

    2) Euryprospic

Leptoprospic face is long and narrow and has a convex profile, prominent upper jaw and small and retracted lower jaw (Retrognathia). In addition, the forehead has a steep slope and the upper edges of the eyeball are prominent and the forehead sinuses are large. The bridge of the nose is long and the eyes are close together (almost similar to the Italians). Euryprospic face is wide. The upper part of the face has less protrusion than the previous type. The forehead is straight, vertical, onion-shaped, and the upper edge of the eyeball is indistinct and the forehead sinuses are small. In addition, the nose is shorter and the eyes are further apart. The cheeks are more prominent and the jaws are forward.

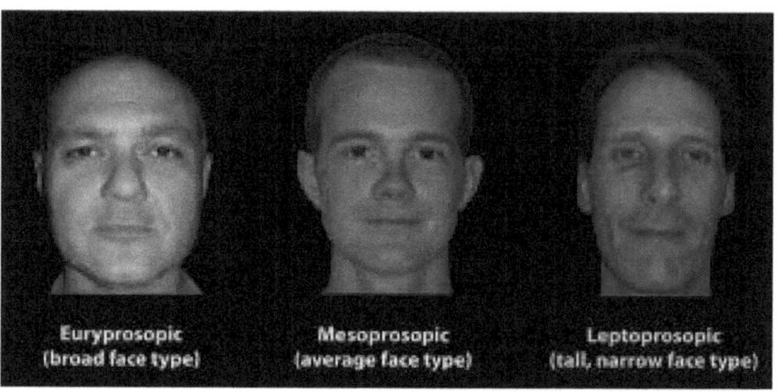

Figure 14. Types of face shapes

The faces show ethnic diversity. In this part, race means the existence of clear characteristics in a group of people. Of course, there is no pure race in man, and in fact there may be diversity. But some features within a group are more than other groups. However, there are usually four ethnic groups:

Negroid race: Usually have Leptoprospic faces that have a prominent upper jaw and mostly thicker and more prominent lips.

Mongoloid: They have a Euryprospic face with a protruding mandible, a vertical forehead, prominent cheekbones, the upper edge of the eyeball, and small frontal sinuses. The cheeks and eye area may be filled with fat sacs. The medial canthus is covered by a skin fold called the epicanthal fold.

Caucasoid race: Most white people, including Iranians, are of this race.

Australoid race: These two have many features in common.
There are also differences between men's and women's faces. Of course, the shape of the face at a young age in girls and boys are similar. Women 's faces reach adulthood earlier than men.

Bony landmarks of the face

Frontal eminence

The area with the most convexity is on both sides of the front of the head, which is about 3 cm above the midpoint of each of the upper sides of the eyeball (Superior orbital margin). These bumps are more pronounced and prominent in women.

Superciliary arch

The smooth, round protrusion is above the inner half of the eyebrow, which is more prominent in men.

Between eyebrows (Glabella)

The bulge in the midline between the two eyebrow arches and above the root of the nose is more prominent in men. This bulge is also the upper level of the eardrum. Due to the high differences between men and women, the forehead is more vertical in women.

Nation

The center of the depression is the root of the nose, which lies below the eyebrows (Glabella) and between the upper two sides of the eyeball, and is actually the junction of the bones of the nose and forehead in the midline.

Orbital margins

The eye socket has four sides, the outer two thirds of which are sharper and smoother. In addition, the medial palpebral ligament and its bony protrusion are felt as a small subcutaneous nodule in the inner corner of the eye. On the outer side, the seam between the forehead bone and the cheekbone (Zygomaticofrontal suture) is palpable as a depression on the outer side of the eyebrow. The lower side of the eyeball is also sharp and palpable.

Supraorbital notch

It is located at the junction of the inner third and the outer two thirds of the upper side and at a distance of 2.5 cm from the midline. If the index finger of one hand is in the middle line, his ring finger indicates this cut. The nerve and arteries of the same name pass through this incision, and if pressure is applied to this nerve, it causes pain. In some people, the incision is closed and perforated. However, applying pressure at this point causes pain. Anesthesiologists use it to stimulate the anesthetized patient.

Infraorbital foramen

This hole is located one centimeter below the lower side of the eyeball and one finger away from the side of the nose. These holes are in a vertical line with the notch above the eyeball and the chin hole. This vertical line crosses the distance between two premolar teeth. From this hole, the arteries and nerves also come out. If you put pressure on this area, the person will feel uncomfortable due to the pressure on the nerve.

Anterior nasal spine

It touches the lower end of the middle septum of the nose (Nasal septum) and the upper lip of the upper lip (Philtrum).

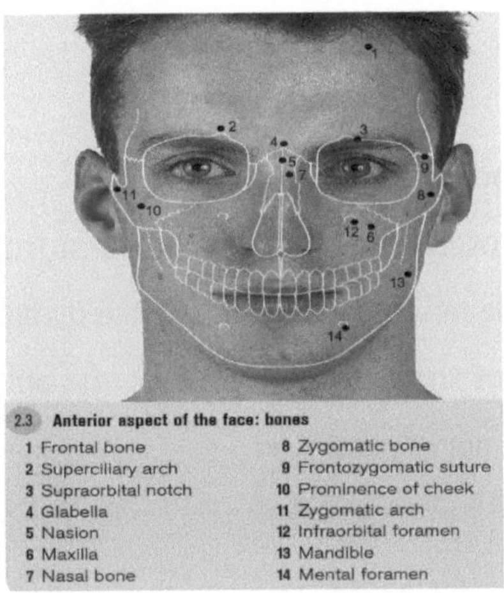

Figure 15. Anterior Aspect of the face

Canine eminence

This protrusion above the canine can be felt from the skin or from inside the vestibule of the mouth and is a sign for dentists to find the hole of the infraorbital foramen. So that the mentioned hole is located above and outside this ridge.

Zygomatic bone

It forms the protrusion of the cheek and can be easily touched and seen.

Jugal point

This point is located at an angle between the arch of the cheekbones and the frontal process of the cheekbones and is palpable.

Zygomatic arch

It is a bony ridge located between the tragus and the earlobe and is easily palpable. It is better to move the fingers from bottom to top to touch the arch.

Articular tubercle root protrusion

When the mouth is closed, this bulge is located in front of the head of the mandible, but when the mouth is open, it is located above it. This protrusion is a superficial sign of the foramen ovale of the sphenoid bone through which the mandibular nerve passes.

Head of mandible

The earlobe is located in front of the tragus and moves under the hand by opening and closing the mandible.

Neck of mandible

It can be felt in front of the earlobe (Lobule) and below the head of the mandible.

Angle of mandible

It is located between the body and the mandible and can be easily touched and seen. This angle is also the level of the second cervical vertebra (C_2) and is smaller (sharper) in men than women.

Base of mandible

Easy to touch. The body of the mandible is also felt from inside the mouth.

Symphysis menti

It touches the midline and has two chin protrusions on both sides of the midline.

Mental foramen

At a distance of 2.5 cm from the midline and the width of one finger above the lower side of the mandible is located between the two teeth of Asia Minor (Premolar). The nerves and arteries of the same name come out of this hole, and the pressure on the hole can be painful.

Coronoid process of mandibular bone

This appendage and the front of the lower jaw (Ramus) are touched from inside the mouth. The back of the mandible is easily touched under the skin.

Maxillary tuberosity

It is felt from the inside of the mouth at the end of the third molar. This sign is used for injections in dentistry.

Mastoid process

It can be easily touched behind the ear.

Styloid process

Between the mandible and the mammary gland (one centimeter inside the mammary gland) just below the outer cartilage of the ear may be palpable.

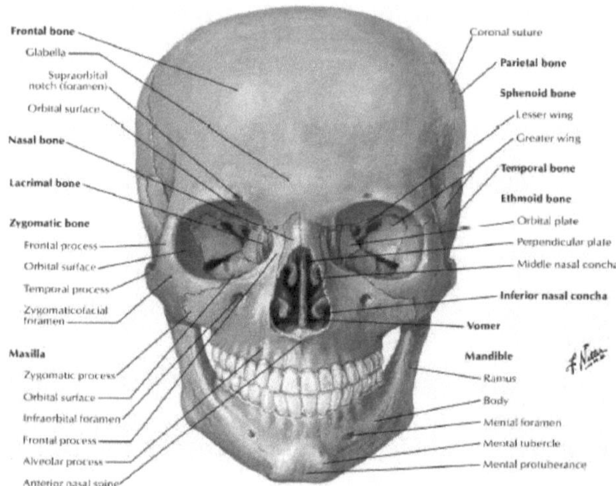

Figure 16. Facial bones

Non-bone signs of the face

Philtrum

It is a depression that extends from the upper lip to the middle septum of the nose (nasal septum).

Red border line (Red border line = Vermilion border)

It is a human characteristic that separates the mucus inside the lips from the skin of the lips.

Nasolabial groove

The upper lip separates from the cheek and extends from the outside of the nasal fin to the corner of the mouth and becomes more pronounced with age.

Buccal fat pad

It is located between the Buccinator and Masseter muscles and atrophies in aging and malnutrition, causing the cheekbones.

With age, other skin folds are found on the face. For example, the under-eye creases form the eye bags, and the outer surface of the corner of the eye forms crevices. These folds are due to the weakening of the skin's connection to the bones and muscles under it, as well as the reduction of elastic fibers in the skin.

Facial expression muscles

They are muscles that are innervated by the facial nerve and are located around the nose, mouth, eyes and ears and change the shape of the face. Their final connection (Insertion) is to the skin. Here are some of the muscles that can be used or examined in superficial anatomy:

Orbicularis occuli

It has three parts: Palpebral, Orbital and Lacrimal. The eyelid is responsible for closing the eyelid gently, and when blinking, the movement is so fast that the person is usually unaware of the muscle action. This part is responsible for the flow of tears on the eyeball and if it is paralyzed, the eyelid will not close and the eye will dry out. The lacrimal part, which is part of the eyelid, is attached to the lacrimal sac and causes tears to be sucked into the nose. The part of the eyeball closes the eye with force.

Precision muscle (Procerus)

This muscle brings the eyelids closer together, and this muscle contracts when you look at bright light.

Corrugator supercilli

It is the only muscle that stretches if a crease is created. This pulls the eyebrow muscle down.

Frontalis muscle

This muscle is actually the anterior ventricle of the occipitofrontalis muscle, which raises the eyebrows and creates a transverse crease in the forehead and prevents sweat from entering the eyes.

Levator labii supperioris alaeque nasi

Raises the upper lip and nasal fins.

Nasal muscle (Nasalis)

It has two transverse parts (Compressor) and a blade (Alar) or dilator that narrows the transverse part of the nasal entrance and widens the part of the entrance feathers. The operation of the second part is more evident in hot weather and in people with shortness of breath.

Depressor septi

It dilates the nostrils by lowering the nasal septum.

Buccinator muscle

It is the muscle that controls the cheek and prevents food from accumulating between the teeth. It is therefore important in dental hygiene. This muscle is also used for whistling and smiling.

Levator and depressor anguli oris muscles

The first raises the corner of the mouth and identifies the teeth when smiling, and the second lowers the corner of the mouth when sad.

Levator labii superioris

It pulls the upper lip upwards and exposes the upper jaw teeth, and also plays a role in the formation of the nasolabial-lip groove.

Depressor labii inferioris

Pulls the lower lip down in times of sadness and doubt.

Zygomaticus major

He raises the corner of his mouth up and out while laughing.

Mentalis muscle

It creates wrinkles in the chin and also turns the lower lip outwards.

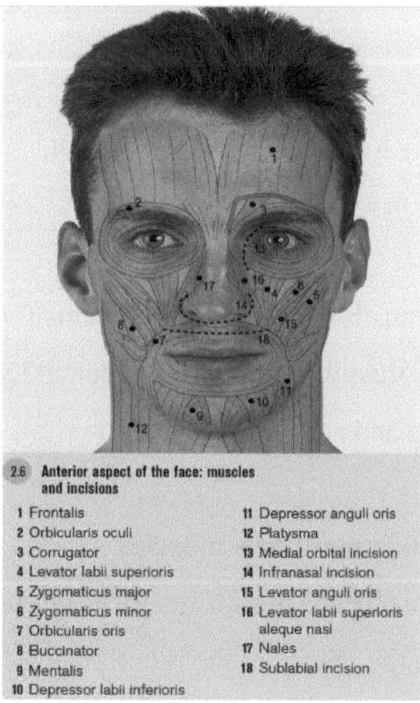

Figure 17. Anterior view of facial muscles

Orbicularis oris annular muscle

He closes his lips and brings them forward. In the corner of the mouth where the different muscles meet, there is a column of tendons (Tendineus) called the axis (Modiolus) that in the corner of the mouth may be felt as a point of stiffness.

It should be noted that facial muscles work in groups and it is not possible to accurately assess the function of a muscle. In addition, the muscles around the mouth are involved in speaking.

Ear muscles (Auricularis)
They attach to the eardrum and in some people the ability to move the ear develops.

Mastication muscles
There are four main masticatory muscles, two of which are palpable or visible in superficial anatomy. All masticatory muscles are innervated by the mandibular nerve.

Temporalis muscle
Clenching and placing your hands on the temples can be felt by touching the muscle fibers under the hand. In addition, when chewing food, the movement of the temporalis muscle can be seen by looking at the migraine area.

Masseter
The lower jaw bone can be touched by pressing the teeth together. Part of the muscle is covered by the parotid gland, but the front side is easily palpable.

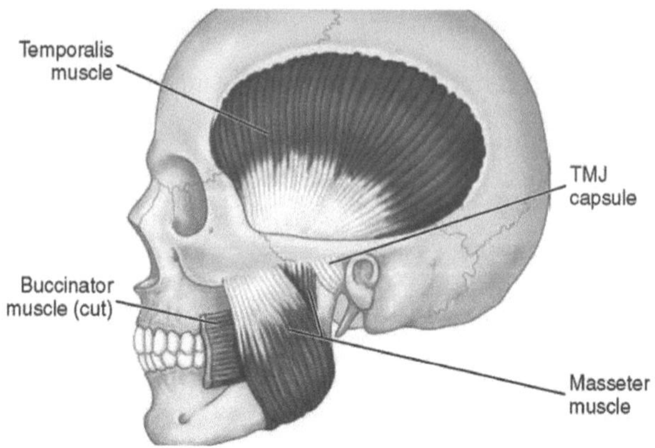

Figure 18. Chewing muscles

Visible buildings and touch on the face

Eye

There are structures in the eye that are visible or palpable in superficial anatomy:

Eyelids (Eyelids = Palpebrae)

The upper eyelid is larger than the lower eyelid. It is covered on the outer surface by the skin and on the inner surface by the conjunctiva. The structure of the eyelid, in addition to the muscles, consists of a connective tissue called the tarsal plate, which forms the main skeleton of the eyelid. This screen can be touched by holding the eyelid between the fingers. The front side of the eyelid has eyelashes on the outside, and there are more rows of eyelashes on the upper eyelid. One-sixth of the inner eyelid does not have eyelashes. The distance between the two eyelids is called the palpebral fissure.

Normally, the upper eyelid slightly covers the symmetry, but the lower eyelid is tangential to the area connecting the symmetry to the sclera. Attached to the upper eyelid is the levator palbebrae superioris. This muscle receives nerves from the third pair of oculomotor nerves, and if this muscle is paralyzed, the eyelid collapses (Ptosis).

Corner or angle of the eye (Canthus)

In the inner corner of the eye, the eyelids are farther apart, and this angle is round, and there is a small space in the inner corner that forms the lacrimal lake, which appears on the surface of the protrusion called the lacrimal caruncle. Just outside of this is a Chinese protrusion of the conjunctiva called the semilunar fold, which acts as the third eyelid in some animals.

Tear point (Punctum lacrimalis)

Between one inner sixth and five outer sixths, each eyelid is a prominent point that removes tears from the eye and transmits them to the tear sac.

Conjunctiva

It is a mucous membrane that covers the surface inside the eyelid and on the sclera. Or sclera and located below the conjunctiva is visible and by looking at the inner surface of the eyelid conjunctiva can be diagnosed anemia. Eye drops are also usually poured into the upper conjunctival obstruction.

Limbus

The junction of the cornea to the sclera is called.

Iris and Pupil

The color plate behind the symmetry is called the iris, which varies from blue to black depending on the amount of pigment. The hole in the middle of the iris is called the pupil, which narrows in response to light. Using an ophthalmoscope and through the pupil, the lens, retina, blind spot (Optic disc) and yellow spot (Macula lutea) can be examined.

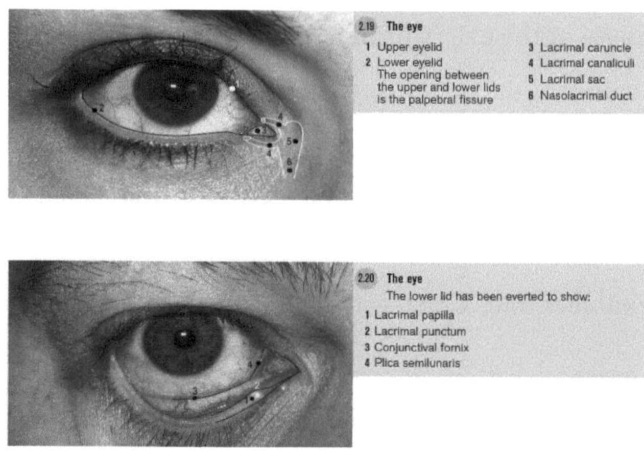

Figure 19. Anatomy of the eye

Nose

The upper part of the nose is made of bone and the lower part is made of cartilage.

Nasal bridge

It is the bony part of the nose that is formed by two nasal bones and is broken in blows to the face.

Greater alar cartilage

Each is C-shaped and is located in the nostril. At the tip of the nose, the groove between the two cartilages is palpable and sometimes visible. The end of this cartilage inside the nasal cavity can be touched with a finger in the form of a ridge.

Vestibule

The part of the nose that is covered with coarse and coarse hair (Vibrissea). Under the skin of the atrium is the nasal septum, which has a large network of vessels called the Kisselbach's plexus. Which is responsible for most of the nosebleeds (Epistaxis).

The profile of a woman's nose is concave to straight, while in men it is straight to convex.

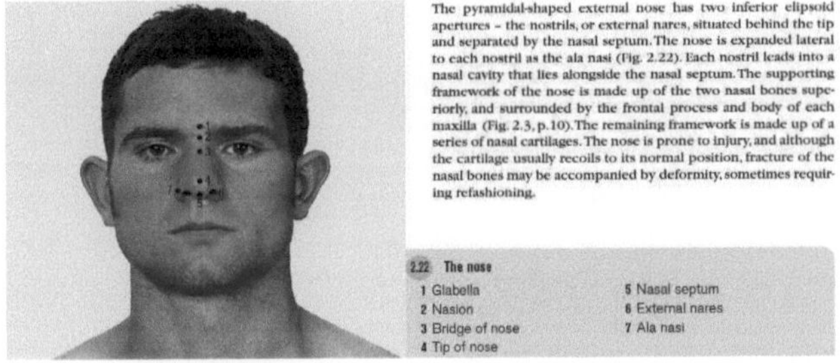

Figure 20. Superficial anatomy of the nose

Paranasal sinuses

There are four pairs of air sinuses in the bones around the nose that lead through the duct to the nasal cavity. In this section, the superficial anatomy of the two frontal and maxillary sinuses, which are more prone to inflammation, is examined.

Frontal sinus

It escapes in the depth of the superciliary arch. To determine its superficial anatomy, it is obtained by connecting the following points of a triangle that defines the boundaries of the frontal sinus:

A) Nasion

B) Centimeter above Nasion in the midline

C) The junction of the inner third and the outer two thirds of the upper side of the eyeball

By pressing under the eyebrows upwards on each side, the sensitivity of the frontal sinuses can be searched.

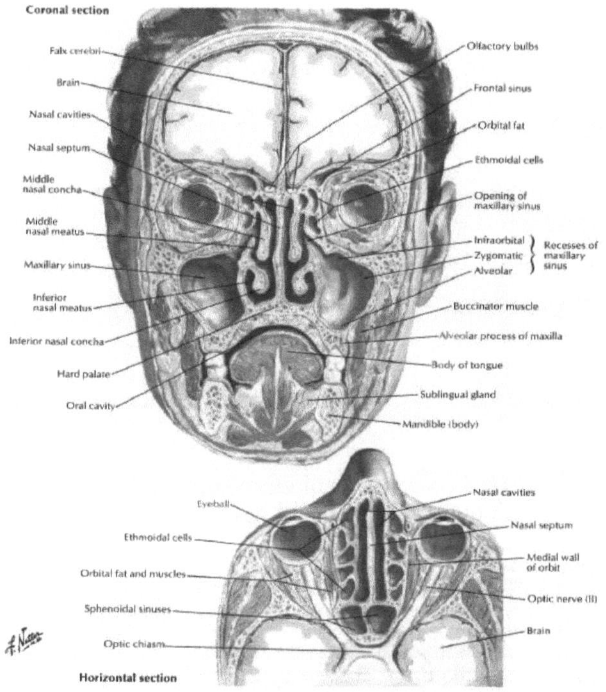

Figure 21. Cross-sectional anatomy of the face

Maxillary sinus

It is the largest air sinus and it is called Higmore antrum cave. It is obtained by connecting the following points of a quadrilateral that characterize the maxillary sinus:

A) One centimeter inside the ridge of the cheekbones just below the lower side of the eyeball

B) One centimeter above and two centimeters behind the angle of the mouth

C) one centimeter above the angle of the mouth

D) Just below the inner end of the lower side of the eyeball

To examine this sinus, place your hand under and inside the cheek and press up.

Mouth

By opening the mouth, the following buildings are seen and touched inside the mouth:

Frenelum of lip

The crease is the mucus that connects the lips to the gums.

Palatoglossal fold = Anterior pillar

The crease is the mucus that separates the throat from the mouth. Behind this crease and below the soft palate, the palatine tonsil can be seen. Of course, in old age, the tonsils become atrophic and not well defined, but in young people, especially when they have a cold, the tonsils look like almonds on the back of the tongue below the palate.

Small tongue (Uvula)

At the dorsal end, the roof of the mouth is seen in the midline and moves by saying the word oh, which can be used to assess the vagus nerve.

The dorsal surface of the tongue

On the dorsal or upper surface of the tongue, the taste buds, and especially on the back of it, are marked circular papillary villi (Circumvalate papilla). Normally, the color of the tongue is pink because the mucous layer on it is thin, but in the disease, the creatine layer of the tongue becomes white (pregnant) due to thickening.

Frenulum of tongue

It raises the tongue to the underside of the tongue, which connects the tongue to the floor of the mouth.

Deep lingual vein

It is a blue protrusion outside the tongue and is marked.

Plica fimbriata

The crease is a mucus located outside the deep vein of the tongue that extends from the floor of the mouth to the tip of the tongue.

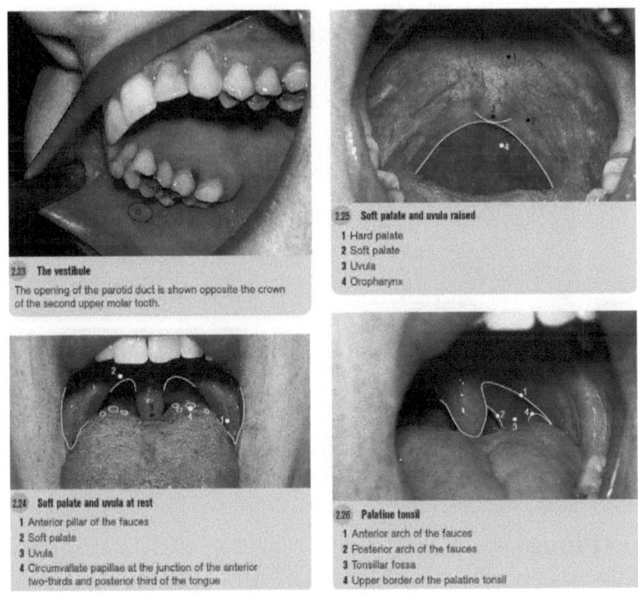

Figure 22. Surgical anatomy. Oral surface

Sublingual papilla

In the palm of the mouth on both sides of the tongue can be felt and seen. The submandibular duct opens and a hole may be seen.

Sublingual fold

The crease is transverse to the floor of the mouth, caused by the placement of a sublingual salivary gland that is easily palpable and visible.

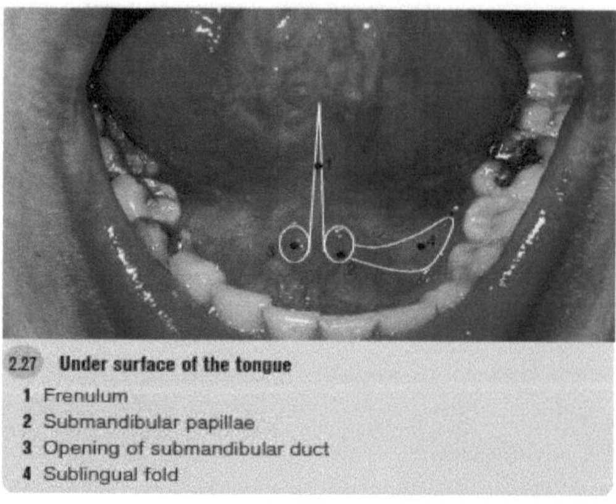

Figure 23. Under surface of the tongue

External ear (Pinna)

The outer ear is made up of a flexible fibrous-cartilaginous piece called the auricle and the outer ear canal. At the end of the external ear canal is the tympanic membrane. In this section, various structures of the external ear that can be touched and observed and used in superficial anatomy are examined.

Lobule of auricle

It consists of fibrous tissue and fat.

Helix

It is a raised edge that starts at the soft end of the ear and ends at its column (Crus of helix) above the outer ear canal. At the top and outside there is a ridge called the Tubercle of Darwin.

Antihelix

This ridge is parallel to Helix and in front of it. This protrusion at the upper end is divided into two columns (Crus) at the top and bottom, which is located between these two triangular spaces (Triangular fossa).

Boat space (Scaphoid fossa)

It is the depression between Helix and Antihelix.

Antitragus

Located at the bottom end of Antihelix.

Tragus

It is a bulge located in front of the outer ear canal and hair usually grows on it in the elderly.

Intertragic notch

It is located between Tragus and Antitragus, which indicates the surface of the jugular foramen.

Concha

It is a space surrounded by Antihelix that leads to the external ear canal.

Cymba concha

It is the space that is created between the Crus of helix and the Inferior crus of antihelix and is located in the depth of the cavity of the upper triangle of the external ear canal (Suprameatal or Macewens triangle), which defines the outer surface (Mastoid antrum).

External acoustic meatus

The duct is S-shaped and 3 cm long. To examine the tympanic membrane or drop ear drops in adults, the eardrum should be pulled up and back and in children down and back. The tympanic membrane and the inside of the middle ear can be examined with an otoscope.

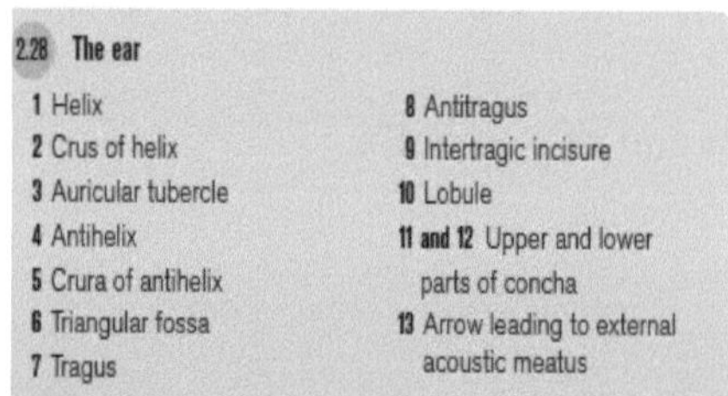

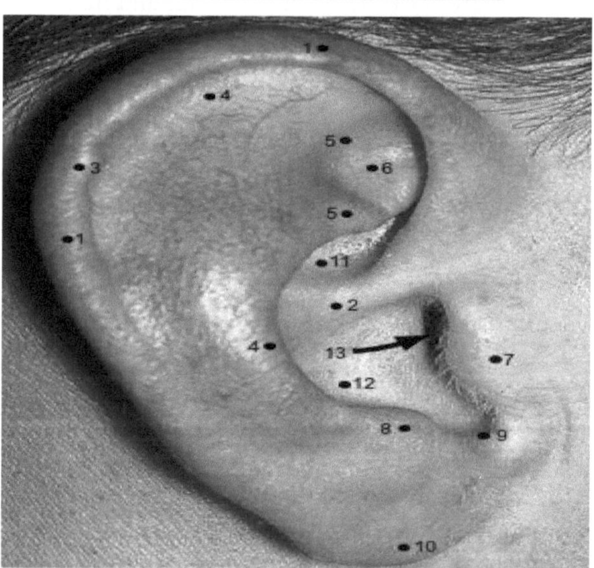

Figure 24. Superficial anatomy of the ear

Parotid gland

It is the largest salivary gland, located between the arch of the cheekbone, the mastoid process, the temporal bone, and the mandible. To determine its surface anatomy by connecting the points below its range is obtained:

A) The head of the mandible

B) Masseter muscle center

C) Two centimeters below and behind the angle of the mandible

D) Masteoid process

The upper pole is located behind the cartilage of the external ear canal and the temporomandibular joint (TMJ) capsule. This pole is slightly concave. The lower pole is round and is located below and behind the angle of the lower jaw. The gland is not easily touched, and if it can be easily touched, it may indicate disease or the small lymph nodes on the ear canal may be swollen. The facial nerve, retromandibular vein, and external carotid artery pass through the gland and may be affected by swelling of the gland.

Parotid duct

It passes about 1-1.5 cm below the arch of the cheekbones and parallel to it over the masseter muscle, and after piercing the buccinator muscle in the atrium of the mouth, it opens in front of the second largest tooth of Asia. The surface path of this duct is the middle linear third that connects the following points:

A) On the tragus of the earlobe

B) The midpoint of the line that connects the nasal plume (Nasa lala) to the side of the upper lip.

By clenching the teeth together, this duct can be slid and touched on the masseter muscle. The entrance to the duct of this gland may also be visible as a papilla in the atrium of the mouth.

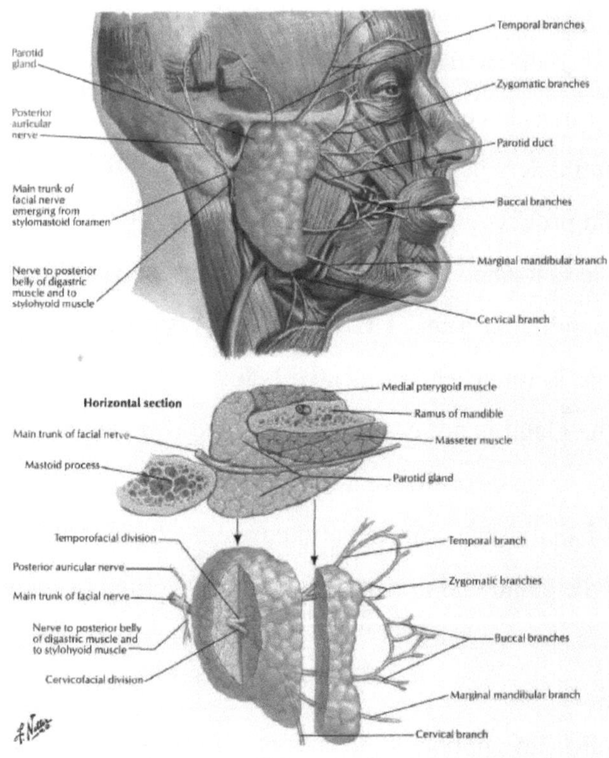

Figure 25. Superficial anatomy and surgery of the parotid gland

Arteries of the Face

Facial artery

In the face, it has a spiral path and is obtained by connecting the points below its path:

A) Next to the front of the masseter muscle on the base of the mandible

B) One centimeter at the corner of the mouth

C) The inner angle of the eye

The pulse of this artery can be felt along the front of the masseter muscle by pressing the teeth together. In addition, if you hold the corner of the lip with one finger inside the mouth and the other finger outside the corner of the lip, you may feel the pulse of the artery. In these places, the artery can be compressed during bleeding and bleeding can be prevented.

Superficial temporal artery

It is one of the two terminal branches of the external carotid artery and its surface path is obtained by connecting the following points:

A) The back of the neck of the mandible on the gland of the earphone

B) Tragus anterior entrance to the arch

C) 5 cm above point b

At point C, it is divided into front and back branches. The pulse of the artery can be felt on the arch of the forearm in front of the tragus and the pulse of the anterior branch on the migraine, or the artery can be pressed at these points to prevent bleeding.

Maxillary artery

It is another terminal branch of the external carotid artery and goes from the depth of the horn (Ramus) of the mandible to the depth of the infratemporal fossa and is determined by connecting the points below its surface path:

A) Anterior earlobe at the level of the mandibular neck

B) Just behind the jugal point, this is a deep artery and its pulse cannot be easily touched.

Middle meningeal artery

This branch separates from the maxillary artery and enters the skull. Extradural haemorrhage. By connecting the following points, its surface path is determined:

A) Intermediate point and arc

B) Two centimeters above point A

The frontal branch of this artery goes from point B to the Pterion and then to the distance between the Nasion and the Inion, and its parietal branch goes to the Lambda.

Supraorbital artery

It is an ophthalmic branch of the eye artery, and its pulse may be palpated about 2.5 cm from the midline at the top of the eyeball.

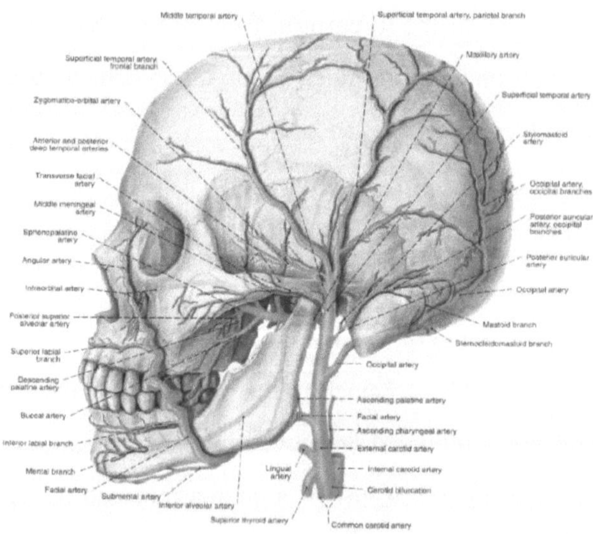

Figure 26. Facial blood vessels and their surgical and superficial anatomy

Veins of the Face

They are almost the same path as the arteries, but slightly different. For example, the facial vein is not spiral and is behind the artery.

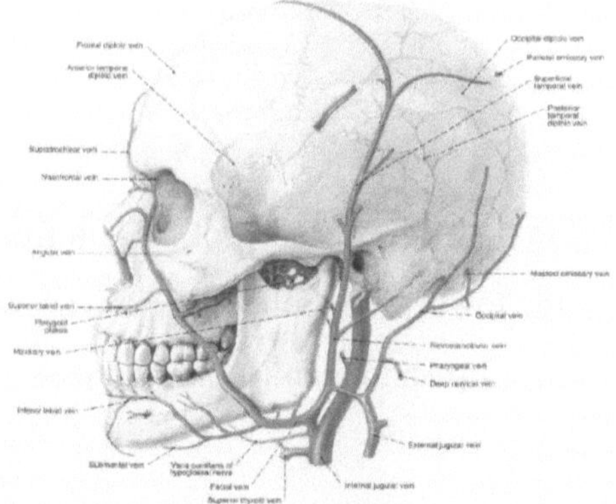

Figure 27. Facial blood supply veins and their surgical and superficial anatomy

Nerves of the Face

Supraorbital nerve

It comes out of the incision above the eyeball. It exits at a distance of 2.5 cm from the midline or 3 fingers from the midline so that one finger in the midline and the third finger represents this nerve. This nerve hurts if you press on this point, and anesthesia can be injected at this point. This nerve gives nerve to the skin of the forehead, and the upper eyelid.

Infraorbital nerve

It protrudes from the hole under the eyeball one centimeter below the lower edge of the eyeball and one finger away from the outside of the nose. At this point, if it is pressed, it hurts and the nerve can be anesthetized at this point.

It can also be anesthetized through the atrium outside the canine eminence. This nerve gives the nerve to the upper lip and lower eyelid. By injecting anesthetic into the hole under the eyeball, the front teeth of the maxilla may also be anesthetized.

Mental nerve

It comes out of the chin hole at a distance of 2.5 cm from the midline and one centimeter above the lower side of the mandible and gives nerves to the skin of the chin and lower lip and it can be anesthetized at this point.

Auricullotemporal nerve

From the back of the temporomandibular joint (TMJ), it travels across the superficial temporal arteries and supplies nerves to the temples, earlobes, and outer scalp. To anesthetize this nerve, anesthesia can be injected in front of the tragus and slightly behind the superficial temporal artery.

Lingual nerve

It passes through the space behind the third molar of the mandible and at this point this nerve can be anesthetized inside the mouth. This nerve is a branch of the mandibular nerve and provides the general sense of two-thirds of the front of the tongue. Its surface path is determined by connecting the following points:

A) Just below the root button of the articular tubercle

B) Two centimeters above the lower side of the mandible in the distance between the angle of the mandible and the symphysis menti

C) Just below the angle of the mouth

Inferior dental nerve

It is a branch of the mandibular nerve that gives nerve to the mandibular teeth and eventually emerges from the canal hole as the canine nerve. Its surface path can be determined by connecting the following points:

A) Just below the Articular tubercle button

B) The center point of the mandible (Ramus) of the mandible

C) Mental foramen

To anesthetize this nerve, anesthesia can be injected slightly behind the anterior side of the mandible.

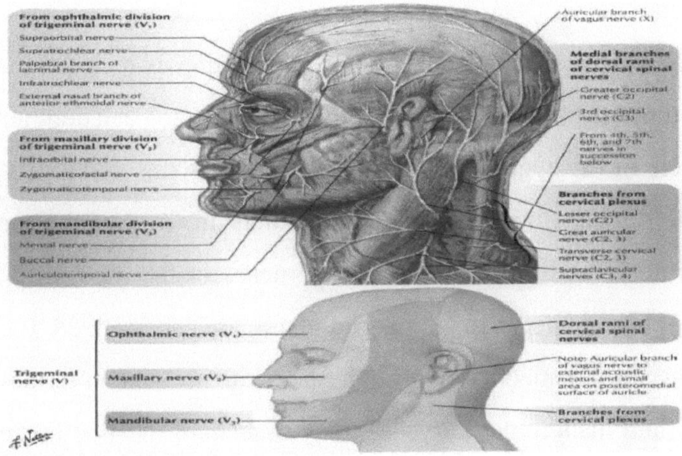

Figure 28. Superficial anatomy of the nerve distribution of the face and neck

Maxillary Nerve

The second branch of the fifth pair of nerves is the trigeminal nerve, which supplies nerves to the teeth of the upper jaw and its skin and mucous membranes. The following methods are used to anesthetize this nerve:

A) By inserting the needle obliquely from the mandibular notch in the front of the mandible head forward and in the Sphenopalatine cavity

B) By inserting a needle into the Greater palatine foramen in the roof of the mouth. This hole is located one centimeter inside the third molar.

C) By inserting a needle through the atrium behind the third teeth of the maxilla.

D) through the atrium of the mouth by inserting a needle into the hole of the infraorbital foramen outside the canine eminence, in which case the whole nerve may be anesthetized.

Mandibular nerve

The third branch is the trigeminal nerve, and a butterfly bone protrudes from the skull through a round foramen. This hole is located at a depth of 4 cm in the tubercle of the zygomotic arch. To anesthetize this nerve, if you insert the needle directly into the mandibular notch, in front of the mandibular head, the nerve and the parasympathetic nerve of the ear (otic ganglion), which supplies the nerve to the parotid gland, are anesthetized. It should be noted that direct injections through the skin are not common for the maxillary and mandibular nerves. In any case, care must be taken that the anesthetic does not enter the veins of the area.

Facial nerve

It is a nerve that has sensory, parasympathetic and motor fibers. After leaving the skull, this nerve enters the parotid gland through the Stylomastoid hole and divides into its terminal branches. The hole is located at a depth of 2 cm in front of the mastoid process. To determine the surface direction of the facial nerve, connect the following points:

A) Antitragus for the ear

B) Right in front of and above the soft earlobe

In fact, the facial nerve pathway is transversely linear and passes through the upper side of the earlobe. This nerve can be found during surgery in front of the SCM muscle at the junction with the mammary gland of the temporal bone just below the external ear canal. After entering the parotid gland, the nerve divides into its last five branches. If you place the heel of the hand on top of the gland and your thumb is in the neck area, the path of the five fingers will show the five terminal branches of the facial nerve in the face, which are:

A) thumb; Temporal branch

B) index finger; Zygomatic branch

C) middle finger; Buccal branch

D) ring finger; Marginal mandibular branch

E) little finger; Cervical branch

In the case of peripheral nerve damage, the muscles of one side of the face (Bell's palsy) paralyze the muscles on the other side of the face and the face is pulled to the opposite side. If the nerve in the brain is damaged (Upper motor neuron lesion), the muscles in the lower part of the face are mainly affected.

Glossopharyngeal nerve

It has sensory, taste, and parasympathetic fibers, and connect the following points to determine its surface path:

A) Right on the anterior surface Intertragic notch earlobe

B) Right in the middle of the mandibular angle

C) Just above the mandible at the junction of the dorsal third and the front two thirds of the mandible

To test this nerve, by stimulating the back of the throat (Gag reflex), the person becomes nauseous.

Nervousness of facial skin

The sensation of the facial skin is mainly innervated by the fifth pair of trigeminal nerves, and only the skin on the parotid gland and the angle of the mandible are innervated by the cervical nerve from the cervical retina.

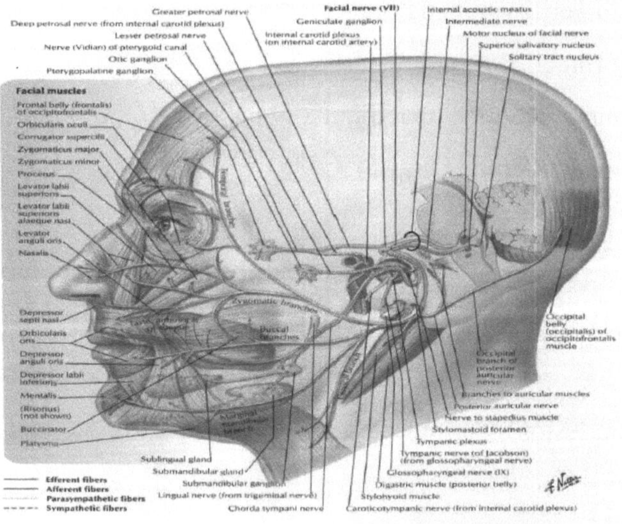

Figure 29. Facial neural distribution

Trigeminal nerve

It has three ocular branches (Ophthalmic, V_1), maxillary (Maxillary, V_2) and mandible (Mandibular, V_3).

Ophthalmic nerve

It innervates the skin of the nose (tip and bridge of the nose), the upper eyelid and the forehead to the scalp (Vertex).

Maxillary nerve

Gives nerves to the skin of the upper lip, nasal fins and skin on the upper jaw and cheekbones.

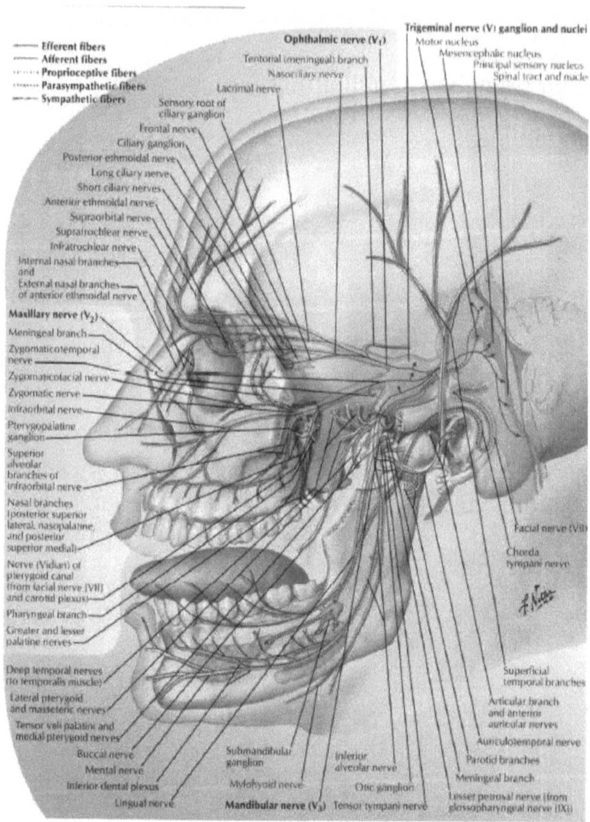

Figure 30. Facial neural distribution

Mandibular nerve

It innervates the skin of the lower lip, chin, upper earlobe, temporal lobe, and skin on the lower jaw except the glands and the angle of the lower jaw.

Great auricular nerve

It is from the cervical network and gives nerves to the skin on the parotid gland and the angle of the mandible.

Nerve of the outer ear

The sensation of the tulip skin and the outer ear canal is provided by several nerves:

Auriculotemporal nerve: Gives nerve to the skin of the upper outer surface and part of the external ear canal.

Great auricular nerve: Gives nerve to the soft skin of the ear and part of the ear canal.

Lesser occipital nerve: Gives nerve to the inner surface (cranial) of the eardrum.

Vagus nerve (sensory branch; Alderman's nerve): Gives nerve to the external ear canal and therefore makes the person nauseous when washing the external ear canal.

Bone signs of cranial roof
Head difference (Vertex)
The highest palpable part of the skull is called.

Frankfurt plane
When standing, the lower sides of the eyeball (Inferior orbital margin) and the upper sides of the external ear canal (External acoustic meatus) are located on a horizontal surface that is used to examine the skull and is known as the Frankfurt surface.

Reid's base line

It is a surface that connects the lower side of the eyeball to the middle of the outer ear canal. This line is clinically important because:

1) Trephination is performed to drain extradural hematoma at this level.

2) The brain (Cerebrum) is located above this level.

3) The cerebellum is located in the lower back third of this surface.

Parietal eminence

It is the most convex part of the parietal bone, which is located on the back, top and sides of the head and is palpable. This bulge is more prominent in women.

Bregma

It is the junction of the frontal and parietal bones, and if you connect the external duct of the two ears with a curved line, the point is 2.5 cm ahead of the midpoint of this line. This point is membranous at birth and is called the anterior fontanelle. This mortar closes up to 18 months.

Lambda

It is the junction of the occipital and parietal bones and is located about 6 cm above the external protrusion of the occiput (inion). At birth, this point is called the posterior fontanelle, which closes at 6 months.

Asterion

It is the junction of the occipital, parietal and temporal bones. This point is about one centimeter above the midpoint of the tragus of the eardrum and the inion.

Sylvian point = Pterion

The junction of the parietal, frontal, temporal, and butterfly bones is H-shaped. This area is about 4 cm above the cheek arch and 3.5 cm behind the frontozygomatic suture. This point is clinically important because:

1) Surface marker of the anterior branch of the middle meningeal artery.
2) The surface marker is the center of the lateral groove of the brain (Sylvian fissure) of the brain.
3) The surface indicator of the islet (Insula) of the brain.
4) It is a superficial indicator of the middle cerebral artery.

Sagittal suture

It stretches between Bregma and Lambda.

Coronal suture

By connecting the Pterion, both sides of its surface path are determined.

Lambdoid suture

By connecting the Asterion on both sides so that it passes through the Lambda, its path is obtained.

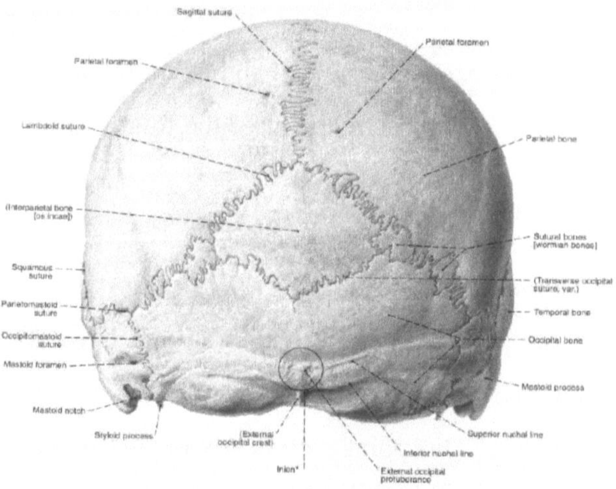

Figure 31. Skull bones and posterior fontanelle

Cranial dural venous sinuses

Superior sagittal sinus

Its surface path is obtained by connecting the following points:

A) Glabella

B) Inion

Straight sinus

If you connect the following points, the surface path is obtained:

A) Two centimeters above the auricle peak

B) External protrusion (Inion)

Transverse sinus (transverse sinus)

Its path is obtained by connecting the following points:

A) Asterion

B) Inion

Sigmoid sinus

By connecting the following points, its surface path is determined:

A) Asterion

B) One centimeter above the tip of the mastoid process (Mastoid process). This sinus is adjacent to mastoid air cells and may become infected or ruptured during infections of these air cells or during surgery.

Cavernous sinus

If you draw a small ellipse one-centimeter-wide and one centimeter above the Articular tubercle, you have determined the surface path of this sinus.

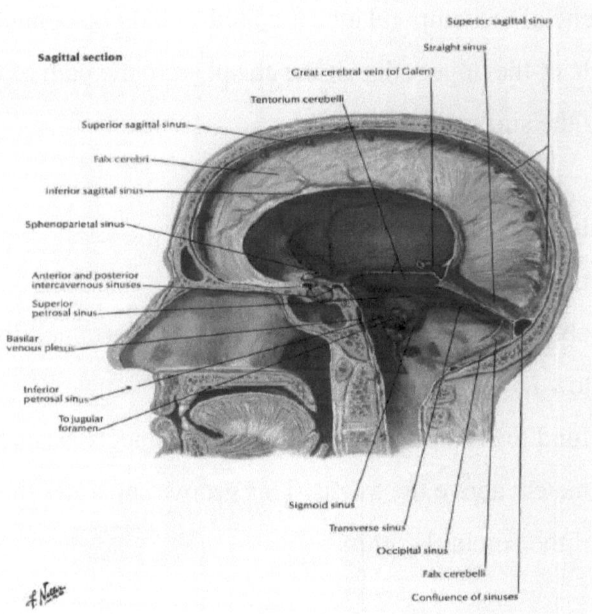

Figure 32. Intracranial venous sinuses

Poles of the cerebrum

Frontal pole

The front end of the lip is called the forehead of the brain and is located slightly above and outside the nasion or below the root of the nose.

Occipital pole

The dorsal end is the posterior lobe of the brain and is located slightly above and outside the inion.

Temporal pole

The anterior end of the temporal lobe is called, and if you connect the pterion and the middle of the upper edge of the cheek arch, the path of this pole will be marked on the surface.

Cerebral Sulci

Central sulcus of Rolando

The frontal lobe separates from the apex and is determined by connecting the points below its surface path:

A) 1.2 cm behind the midpoint of the line that connects Nasion and Inion.

B) Five centimeters above the tragus. This groove separates the sensory and motor areas of the cerebral cortex.

Precentral sulcus

It is 1.25 cm (half an inch) in front and parallel to the central groove. Between this groove and the central groove of the postcentral gyrus is the brain.

Postcentral sulcus

It is located at a distance of 1.25 cm in the back and parallel to the central groove. It is located between this groove and the central groove of the central China.

Lateral sulcus of Sylyius

The temporal lobe separates the frontal and parietal lobes and is centered in the Pterion and has three horns:

Posterior ramus

It is the largest horn and is seven centimeters long and is determined by connecting the points below its surface path:

A) Pterion

B) Two centimeters below the parietal eminence

C) parietal bulge

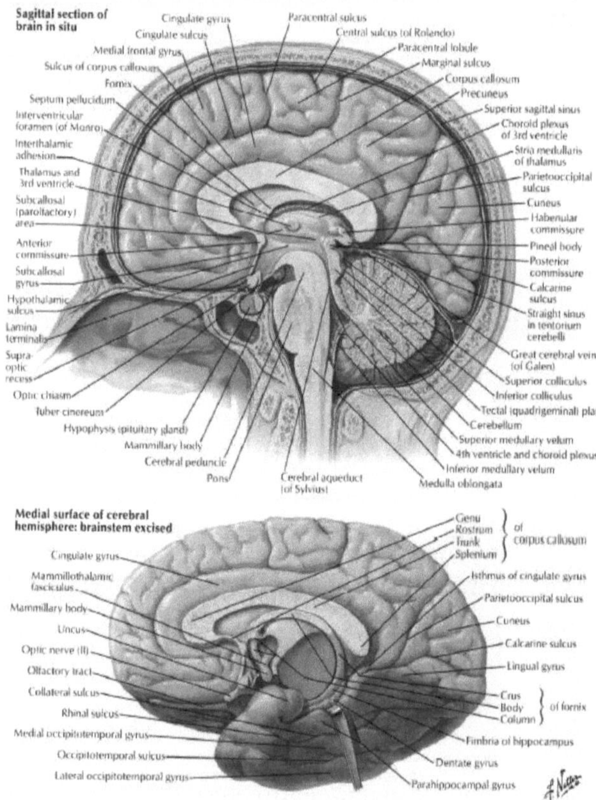

Figure 33. Superficial anatomy and brain surgery

Ascending ramus

If you draw a vertical line two centimeters long from Pterion, its path will be determined.

Anterior ramus

If you draw a line 2.5 meters long from the Pterion transversely and forward, it will determine the path of this horn.

Superior temporal sulcus

If you draw a line at a distance of 1.25 cm and parallel to the lateral horn of the lateral groove, the path of this groove will be determined and the lower temporal groove will be 1.25 cm away from the upper temporal groove and parallel to it.

Parieto-occipital sulcus

If you draw a line 5 cm long from 5 cm above the inion downwards and slightly forward, the path of this groove, which is located at the level inside the cerebral hemisphere, will be determined.

Important areas of the brain (Cortical areas)

Motor area

In China, the precentral gyrus is located between the precentral and central grooves.

Sensory area

In China, the posterior center is the parietal lobe, between the central and posterior grooves.

Acoustic area

In the middle of the upper temporal fold (Superior temporal gyrus) is located between the lateral and upper temporal grooves.

Motor speech area of Broca

The area between the ascending branches and the front of the lateral groove. Damage to this center causes speech impairment (Aphasia).

Visual area

Around the groove (Calcarine) is the occipital lobe, a small area just above the inion.

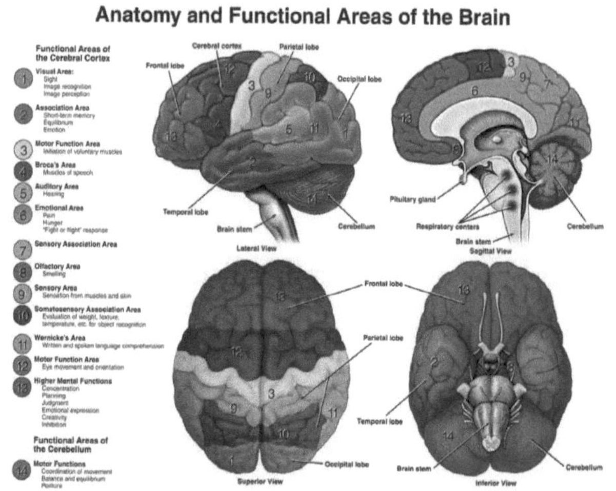

Figure 34. Anatomy and functional Areas of the Brain

References

Halim superficial anatomy

Anatomy of Snell Surgery

Anatomy of Surgery Greys

Surface anatomy

Snell Superficial Anatomy

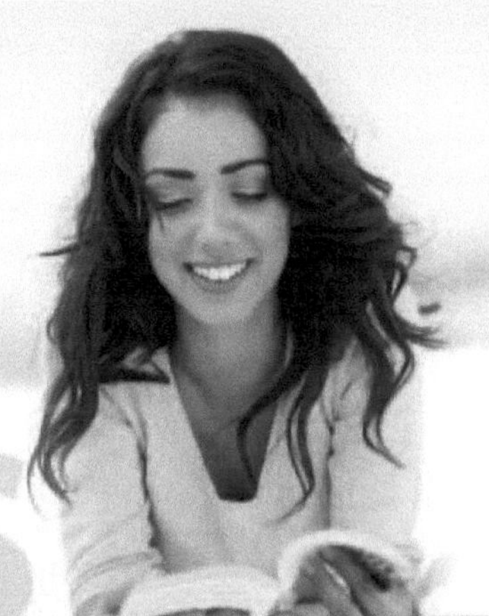

yes I want morebooks!

Buy your books fast and straightforward online - at one of world's fastest growing online book stores! Environmentally sound due to Print-on-Demand technologies.

Buy your books online at
www.morebooks.shop

Kaufen Sie Ihre Bücher schnell und unkompliziert online – auf einer der am schnellsten wachsenden Buchhandelsplattformen weltweit! Dank Print-On-Demand umwelt- und ressourcenschonend produziert.

Bücher schneller online kaufen
www.morebooks.shop

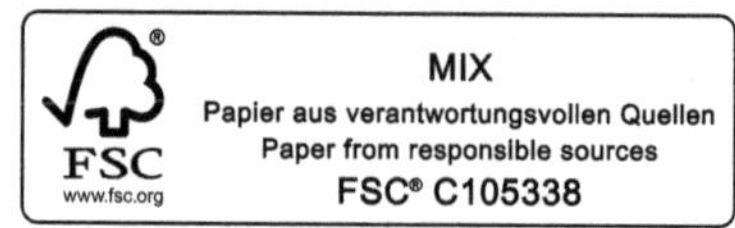

Printed by Books on Demand GmbH, Norderstedt / Germany